Patience FOR THE
PATIENT
"Hope & Healing"

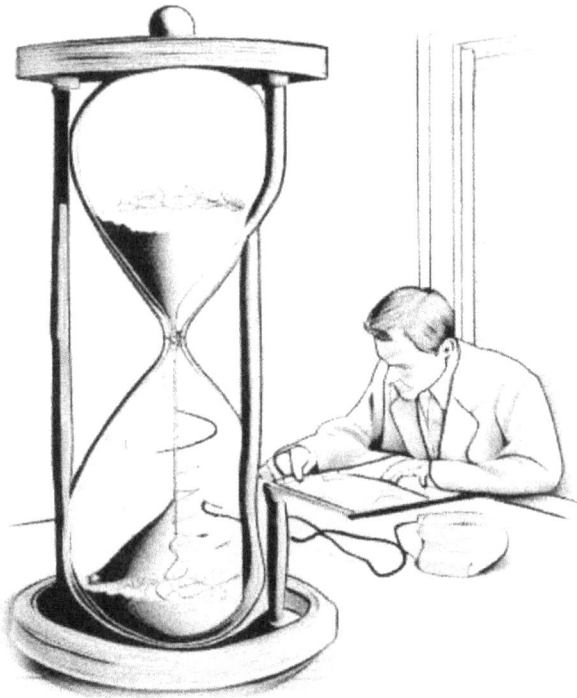

George Hansen & Yvette Kilgore

Illustrations and cover design by Tom Garber

Published by Here I Am Publishing, LLC
780 Monterrosa Drive
Myrtle Beach, South Carolina 29572

HERE I AM
PUBLISHING, LLC

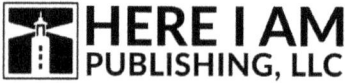

ISBN: 978-1-958032-20-6

This book is dedicated
to those who have given,
those who have received,
and those who continue
to wait for an organ.
May those giving, give freely
in faith; those receiving,
receive with joy; and those
waiting continue to...

Wait well with
hopeful expectation
that their day
is coming.

*"And this hope will not lead to
disappointment. For we know
how dearly God loves us,
because he has given us
the Holy Spirit to fill our
hearts with his love"*
– Romans 5:5 (NLT).

TABLE OF CONTENTS

Acknowledgments - George Hansen

This book would not have been written and published without the help and encouragement of a community of family and friends. These specific family and friends are my community, and I am grateful for their love and support. Specifically, I want to thank my family and friends for supporting me through the donation process even though at times they may have disagreed with my decision. My father, George Hansen, counseled me throughout the decision-making process of becoming a living donor. My stepfather, Jeff Lipman, and mother, Bobbie Lipman, walked with me through the donation surgery and recovery process. And my children, Olivia and London Hansen, helped me through recovery once I returned home. Numerous friends also cared for me throughout my time of recovery, and I am grateful for their continued companionship to this day.

Thank you, Sandi Huddleston-Edwards, for taking the time to listen to my story and idea for this book. Her encouragement to write and share my story alongside Yvette Kilgore means so much to me as a first-time published author. Without Sandi's steadfast support and gentle nudges toward the completion of this book, it would not have been written. Thank you, Yvette Kilgore, for coming alongside me on this journey of expression and discussion of our struggles and triumphs through the living organ donation process. I am grateful for your heart to proceed and your time spent helping to bring our stories to life. Thank you, Yvette's family, for sharing your stories with the world.

The providence of God brought everyone together for the creation of this book, including the doctors, nurses, and living organ donor coordinating staff at MUSC in Charleston, SC. Without their tireless dedication and passion for health and healing, these stories would not exist. Thank you to all living donors who have gone before me and have been a part of improving the process of renewing life within a recipient. Thank you, Doctor Teresa Rice, for tirelessly working to advance organ donation surgery. May you continue to build upon the teachings of your predecessors to further enhance the nephrectomy procedure and bring more healing to more people.

Acknowledgments - Yvette Kilgore

I want to acknowledge all my family and friends who were with Jake, Jason, and me during both transplants. Many were there in person, and all had us in their thoughts and prayed for us through each step of the way. We thank you from the bottom of our hearts and love you for loving us. Your love and faith knowing that God was with us and the doctors and nurses gave us peace and comfort always.

I also acknowledge George Hansen for agreeing to meet with me and be willing to include my input in this book that was in his heart to write to encourage others to consider being an organ donor. It was a pleasure working with you and getting to know you and the wonderful, caring person you are. I am grateful to be able to call you my friend.

And I also acknowledge our friend and publisher, Sandi Huddleston-Edwards, for encouraging us and always being there for us during the process of writing this book. Thank you so much. We could never have accomplished this without you and wish you the best always with your publishing company that is all for God's Glory. You are truly a living servant of our Heavenly Father, and a friend that we are blessed to have in our life.

This is a Spiritual Book...

Yvette and I authored this book because we believe we live this life to be world changers—and we are here to participate and engage with the will of God to be salt and light in Jesus' name. This means we lay down our lives to pick up the life God has for us— believing His plans and purposes are far greater than anything we can think of or imagine.

Yvette writes from the perspective of a mother who has a son who needed a kidney transplant. The need was an unexpected reality placed before her family. With a sense of peace and confidence that God had blessed the path before her, she knew her purpose was to be the donor to her son.

I write from the perspective of one who felt the call to become a living organ donor. I did not wake up one morning deciding to become a living kidney donor; in fact, I didn't know it was an option outside of a family member. The call came, and I answered because I believe in a greater purpose and a higher calling. I could not do this on my own and never would have until my eyes were opened to the need for living organ donors. I was presented with an opportunity to help.

We all may face different situations and circumstances that lead to the need for a transplant. By sharing our experiences and talking with others involved in different ways through the process, by building on God's Word, and by sharing scripture and prayer, our hope is that we can give insight that will give comfort and show compassion, so you know that you are not alone and that with God on our side, all things are possible.

This book is for those considering living organ donation and for those facing an organ transplant. This is also for their families. We want to give hope: hope for a new beginning, hope for restoration, hope for healing, hope for the future and growth in your faith and trust in our Lord. Thoughts and emotions can be overwhelming for a donor and recipient, but may you have comfort knowing others have gone before you and have come through victoriously.

Becoming a living donor is a blessing that can give a patient a chance to receive an organ without being on the waiting list and is something that most of us can do for another person in need. Being a living organ donor is not only a blessing for the recipient, but also a blessing for the donor knowing he/she gave renewed life to someone in need, whether to a relative or a stranger.

We read in Matthew 22:39 (NKJV) that the second great commandment of Jesus is to love your neighbor as yourself. Our neighbors are everyone everywhere! Our willingness to donate an organ to someone in need shows our obedience to this commandment, which is taught to us over and over throughout the Bible. The need for living organ donors is great, and we pray that you will consider being tested to see if you might be the one to fill that need for your neighbor.

The causes and reasons that people may need transplants can be so vastly different. There are genetic conditions that can be the reason one is needed or physical injuries or a heart defect. Also, chronic conditions, such as diabetes, can also cause a person to need some type of organ transplant. The different circumstances are numerous. Not only heart or liver or kidney transplants are needed at times, but also lung, pancreas, and small intestine transplants are needed by men, women, and children for many varied reasons. The most needed and most transplanted organ though are the kidneys. According to the National Kidney Foundation, one in three Americans are at-risk for kidney disease.

According to the UNOS (United Network for Organ Sharing), "6,466 people became living donors in 2022, fewer than 2021." And also, "The need is real. Another person is added to the waiting list every nine minutes." Educate yourself with all the information available out there now on becoming a living donor.

Cast of Characters...

GEORGE HANSEN

George Hansen is the father of two beautiful and loving daughters. George's life centers around his family and faith in Jesus as Lord and Savior. George believes in leading by example and loves helping people. In 2020, George was inspired to begin the process of becoming a living kidney donor. George was approved to donate in 2021 and had surgery in 2022. Even though his donation has been given, George believes the work continues to encourage others to become living donors. He also loves to encourage those who are waiting for a donation as well. George and Yvette met not long after his donation surgery and decided to share their stories together in this book that will hopefully help give patience to the patient in need.

BOBBIE LIPMAN

Bobbie is the mother of George Hansen. She shares in this book about her experience as being a family member of someone who desires to become a living donor. She talks about her initial thoughts when her son shared about his interest in becoming a donor and how she wrestled with accepting the idea. Throughout this book you will read about her expressions of love and concern for the health and well-being of her son as she walked alongside him throughout the living organ donation process. She hopes family members in similar situations will find comfort and guidance in her reflections through her first hand witnessing of a son becoming a living organ donor.

YVETTE KILGORE

Yvette is the mother of Jacob (Jake) Kilgore, Jason Kilgore, Lori Kilgore-Benfield, and is the wife of Gary Kilgore. She shares in this book about being the donor to her son, Jake, who needed a kidney transplant in 1994 when he was just 19 years old. She also talks about what it is like to be on the waiting side of a transplant surgery seventeen years after being a donor. Her son, Jake, needed another kidney transplant when the first donated kidney was beginning to be destroyed by the disease that caused the need for his first transplant. His twin brother, Jason, stepped up and donated a kidney to him. Her perspective in different roles as a mother, discovering her son needed a kidney to continue to live, as a donor for her son at that time, and then as a mother years later when both her sons, one a recipient for a kidney and the other the donor, along with her emotions, worries, and then joy of it all being successful, gives much insight into these experiences that she hopes will help someone facing one of these situations.

GARY KILGORE

Gary is Yvette's husband and the father of their three children He shares the emotions of dealing with his son Jake when he needed and received two kidney transplants through the years. He sat for many hours in the waiting room while his wife and one son were in surgery and while a kidney was being harvested from his wife to be transplanted in his son Jake. Even though he was surrounded by family and friends, it was a moment that put him through all kinds of emotions to process. And then again, he sat with his wife and family and friends years later, waiting while both his sons were going through the same surgeries. He was filled again with similar emotions and worries that he shares.

LORI KILGORE-BENFIELD

Lori is Gary and Yvette's daughter and Jake and Jason's sister She was a new wife in 1994 when her brother first had to have a kidney transplant. She has always been very close to her brothers and her parents, and it was a difficult time to cope with first her mother and brother Jake, being in the operating room at the same time for such a serious operation, and then again years later when both her brothers were in there at the same time for the same surgery. Always seeing her brothers as healthy teenagers and grown men was a challenging thing to handle for her since she never thought something like that would happen in her immediate family—especially when her brother seemed so healthy from the outside. She shares her emotions and experiences in hopes of helping others who may face this journey in life.

JASON KILGORE

As the twin brother of Jake, of course, they are close in every way. They shared all experiences in life together along the way: being infants, learning new things, attending school years, participating in sports together, especially mountain biking and soccer, and just enjoying life as close brothers. Growing up, he never imagined that his seemingly healthy brother would one day be in a position where he needed someone to offer him one of his/her kidneys, so he could continue living a good life. Jason was there for the first transplant in 1994 and worried about his mother and brother. When another kidney was needed for Jake in 2013, there was no doubt in his mind that he would be the one to give it to him. Of course he would! The strong brotherly love they shared made it a "no brainer," as he said. Like the others, he can share his experience about being on different sides of this type of surgery with others too.

JACOB (JAKE) KILGORE

Jake does not hesitate to share that he knows how blessed he has been to have such a loving and devoted family who has always been there for him and given him many more years to be on this earth. These transplants helped ensure he would be able to watch his son, Liam, grow up and become the loving and caring young man he is today. Things were not always easy for Jake during the years he was sick before needing a second transplant, but it did not stop him from always being thankful and patient, knowing that he had a great support system through it all and that his faith would get him through each time. Jake shares his viewpoint through both surgeries and how they were different in many ways each time. First as a 19-year-old when he was young and had his whole life ahead of him and then again at 36-years-old. He was a father to a young son that he wanted to be there for through his life. You will not hear him complain, but he will give some insight into the different thoughts and feelings he went through during the uncertain times of each transplant. Yes, he worried about his mother and then his brother. He was putting them in some danger of doing this for him, but because of the love they all shared, he knew without a doubt that they would be there no matter what and even do it again if they could. He was blessed beyond measure to have two loving, living donors in his family willing to do this for him. He does not take it for granted.

"Also, I heard the voice of the Lord, saying: 'Whom shall I send, and who will go for Us?' Then I said, 'Here am I! Send me."
– **Isaiah 6:8 (AMP)**

"The Lord is near to all who call on Him, to all who call on Him in truth."
– **Psalm 145:18 (NIV)**

Part 1 - The Call

Yvette:

My first experience and thoughts about organ transplants weren't something I expected might happen in my life. My realization of this need by thousands of people was made aware to me right in my own home. It wasn't until one of my twin sons, Jake, would need a kidney transplant to continue living his life that I began to realize the need that so many people have who are waiting for a transplant.

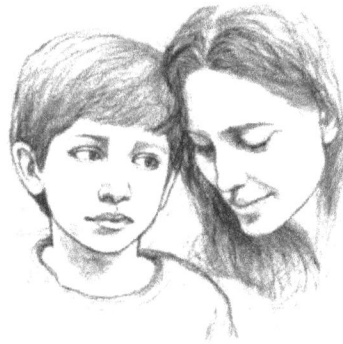

I was shocked and devastated when I found out my 16-year-old son would need a kidney transplant. This was discovered when he and his twin brother had undergone a sports physical required to play on the junior high school soccer team after we moved to Huntersville, NC, from California in 1989.

My husband, Gary, was also completely devastated and thought this could not be happening; there must be something wrong with all this, but there was not. He was very emotional and knew he had to gather himself. He started praying for a miracle.

This was a necessary truth made known to our family that we would never have imagined. Our family was healthy and had no serious illnesses known from our ancestors to alert us of this possibility in one of our children. They were strong, active, happy, and seldom sick so far in life—just a cold here and there—all previous physicals never raised any red flags.

I thought the doctor must have been mistaken when he said our son, Jake, was diagnosed with a disease called IgA Nephropathy (Berger's disease), an incurable disease that can attack the kidneys, causing them to stop functioning and lead to kidney failure for some people. Others diagnosed with this disease may not experience any complications at all, and the disease may even go into remission on its own; however some people develop more complications as the condition progresses, which was the case with Jake.

I went through all the emotions a mother does when she finds out her son has an incurable disease that will require an organ transplant. I was sad, worried, and afraid for him and asked why it was happening to my son that always seemed so healthy. The questions seemed endless in my mind. The quiet disease that had been working in his body for years had been triggered by an unknown source and was now working fast to destroy his kidneys. There had been no symptoms; if it were not for the blood work during the sports physical, we would not have found out when we did.

After the initial shock settled, and I could think more rationally, I could then see what we had to be thankful for. We had to be thankful that this disease was revealed because of the physical. We had to be thankful there was something that could be done for my son, so he would not die. And we had to be thankful that we had been led to this place where CMC (Charlotte Medical Center), now Atrium Health Carolinas Medical Center, had a team of top transplant surgeons on staff.

Through my praise and thanks to God, I saw clearly that I would be the donor to my son when the time came for the transplant. My faith in God and knowing He has always been right beside me all through my life gave me peace and blessed assurance that all would be well. I trusted that He had laid the path before me, and I had no fear. I had always been healthy and taken care of myself, and I felt this was truly God's plan for me to be able to give a kidney to Jake. I believed God was not ready for his life to end yet. He was a kind, caring young man, always wanting the best for others. He had much more kindness to be able to share with others, and I felt I was being allowed to extend that life for him, a second birth if you will, by the grace of God.

We are not promised in life we will not have any battles to face. Satan takes pleasure in our tough times. His plan is to turn us away from Jesus when things do go wrong and convince us to blame God for letting it happen. It is so very easy for us to blame God, to feel He is failing us, and to begin to doubt Him and think it is up to us to make sure things turn out the way we want them to, even when in many cases, there is nothing we can do at all. If we let those thoughts and feelings continue in our minds and hearts, we feel hopeless, like nothing will ever get better, and we lose our faith that life can ever be good again. This is the time to "Let Go, and Let God"; then and only then can we leave room in our minds and hearts for His will to be done in our lives and in our circumstances.

> *"When anxiety was great within me, your consultation brought joy to my soul."*
> **– Psalm 94:19 (NIV)**

Casting our cares is a choice. We must consciously hand over our anxiety to Christ and let Him carry the weight of our concern. He doesn't care if they are little or big concerns. He asks us to turn them all over to Him.

During our times of trials and tribulation, God has not left us. He is patiently waiting for us to come to Him, to repent of our sin of blaming and doubting Him and allow God to do His will in the situation. Instead of being mad at God and feeling like He is letting us down, we need to be praising Him and thanking Him for all He has gotten us through before, and then trust and obey His word that He is with us every step of the way—even in our darkest moments. He will not desert us. We put limits on God when we don't trust in Him.

Proverbs 16:9 says, *"In their hearts humans plan their course, but the Lord establishes their steps"* (NIV). Allow this to happen in your life. His plan is better than anything that we could ever imagine. Trust Him.

Jake:

I noticed more of a change in my endurance and energy during my junior year at North Mecklenburg High School while I was playing on the school soccer team. I just could not keep up as normal when running up and down the field while playing the game.

At first, I was just thinking I was out of shape because I felt healthy and was not aware of anything different going on in my body. I could not really see any reason to be slowing down other than being out of shape or not sleeping well.

After finding out I had a disease attacking my kidneys that would lead to my needing a transplant one day, I was at first in a state of denial thinking it was something I had that could be fixed easily instead of needing a transplant. After all, in my mind, I was a normal strong and healthy 16-year-old guy who felt like I could do everything without any problems. I learned and accepted that was not the case, and I knew it had to be done one day. I had no choice but to roll with it. My faith and my family gave me the love and support I needed to face it head on.

With all the support from family and friends, my faith in God was strengthened, and I felt more connected to Him. Prayer and having access to pray and talk to others whenever and wherever was a great tool to help me cope.

God and the love of my family helped to keep me in control of my emotions and fear. I had a girlfriend at the time who had faith and was incredibly positive about my situation. It was genuinely nice and might have been much different if she had not been there to talk to. I did try to stay positive and eat healthy and exercise. I did not make it a life mission, but I was conscious of it. After all, I was still *me*.

I lived my life as anyone would for my love interest and for the family who had been through it all with me. I kept having fun and doing the things I loved, and I believe that helped to keep me living a *normal* life. I didn't let things I could not control affect me, and it helped to keep me positive and focused on being me.

Lori:

The news did not hit me at first when I heard my brother, Jake, needed a transplant because I saw a young, healthy, handsome junior high school boy who showed no signs of an incurable illness on the outside. But then I saw donor paperwork and information pamphlets lying on the kitchen table for the family to read and BOOM! It hit! This is for real! I learned he only had one functioning kidney, and it was failing too. I just kept thinking, *This cannot be happening to him! This is crazy. My baby brother IS really sick, and his life depends on a transplant! How did this happen?* Fear for him crept in with the "whys?" and "what ifs?"

- *What if none of us are a match?*
- *Why does this have to be happening to HIM?*
- *Is he going to die if we don't find a match?*
- *How long does he have to wait if he needs to be put on a donor list?*
- *What happens after the transplant?*

I honestly had many questions that I don't think I ever asked. Maybe I did not want to know the answers. But, everyone else and I didn't have time to get answers to all the questions, so...OK! Where do I sign up? This is my little brother, and of course, I will be a donor if I am a good match, no question about that! I never would have let Jake or the rest of my family know that I was scared and add to the upset. I just wanted to know what we needed to do to make my brother better and to do it quickly. I didn't want to wait; I felt and knew deep down that I could not lose my brother to this, and it made me so very scared.

Bobbie:

I thought, *Here we go again.* Another idea where my son wanted to offer more than I felt he should, and he overextended himself. At this point in time, he now had his two daughters, my granddaughters, living with him. I felt he needed to focus on them, and the idea of donating a kidney could put them in jeopardy. I mean I could understand if it were a close friend or family member who was in need, but to consider a donation to a complete stranger of this deep and personal level was foreign to me. Please don't misunderstand me. I consider myself a very loving, creative, and generous person. I love to learn new things and challenge myself every day. I worked hard as an educator and fostered the learning of elementary age children for over thirty years. I believe we are on this earth to help one another, especially our families, but this just seemed like too much.

I had an honest expression of my thoughts with my son, and I could tell he had hoped for a positive reaction. But as a mother, I couldn't withhold how I felt about his idea. I love my son, and I want to see him live a long healthy life, and I thought this would be a challenge for him living with one kidney instead of two. I had a lot of worrisome thoughts as I considered his idea of becoming a living kidney donor. *How would his body react? What if there were complications during surgery? How long would he be away from work to recover? What if he needed a kidney years later? My son has enjoyed exercising and staying fit for over ten years. What if he wasn't able to resume exercise after the donation?* As a mother, I didn't want to see my son suffer through something he didn't have to do.

Some of my questions he answered during our discussion. He pointed out that kidney transplant surgeries have been performed for over fifty years. This wasn't an experimental surgery or new procedure. This was a process that had been tested and refined through decades of trial and countless positive outcomes. He told me surgery recovery would take a matter of weeks instead of months, and the incisions were not nearly as large as they used to be years ago. He also said help was available from the National Living Donor Assistance Center to cover the cost of transportation, lodging in Charleston, SC, for testing, and any loss of wages during recovery. I still wasn't comforted much. He was putting his life on the line for someone he had never met and may not ever meet. Even with all the medical advancements and social/economic support, I knew no one could 100 percent guarantee a positive outcome. I didn't want him to proceed, but we both agreed the preliminary testing wouldn't be harmful. At the very least, he would be told he had a healthy body, and his years of running and exercising gave him a lot of benefit, or a hidden sickness would be found, and he could get treatment. Nevertheless, I would have preferred he had walked away from the idea completely. But what could I do other than express my thoughts in hopes he would listen.

George:

 My first thoughts were excitement and wonder. I looked at the sticker on the back of the car in front of me at a red light in Florence, SC, and thought, *What if I am a match?* I called the number on the sticker because I wanted to know. I was curious. A representative from the living kidney donor team at MUSC (Medical University of South Carolina) in Charleston, SC, answered the call. I shared the name I saw on the sticker and how I felt compassion for this person. I wanted to know more about helping him/her. The person on the other end of the phone shared what information she could and said if I would like to continue in the process, I would have to give some blood samples for testing. I said, "Let's go!" Again, I thought, *What if I am a match?* I also asked myself, *What am I getting myself into?* And, *Will this lead to surgery? I have a career and family to support.* I didn't know all the details, but I knew committing to a blood test was the least I could do to help. If I weren't a match, then I could say I tried, and if I were a match, I could praise God for connecting me with this person in need. I knew I had to at least try to help, so I moved forward with excitement and wonder.

 At this point, I didn't even discuss my decision with family or friends because I wanted to wait and see what would happen. I had no idea to what great journey I had been led, but I did know God was with me. Because of my previous life experiences, I knew He would see me through this call. If this call came a few years earlier, I am not sure I would be as confident to make that declaration, but as we grow into the love God has for us as His children through Jesus, we see more and more how on time He is and how faithful He is to lead us through the challenges and calls of life.

 The Bible says, "The just shall live by faith," and I wholeheartedly believe this truth. Our Creator, our Father in Heaven, our God does not call us to live by our good works, but He calls us to live by faith in Him and the finished work of Jesus Christ.

From the moment of Adam through the end of Revelation, we can see, "The just shall live by faith." God desires for us to trust in Him and submit to His ways, plans, and purposes because the life we live on this earth is more than just living for ourselves. God wants us to participate in His purposes. We are here to make a positive difference and be influencers in faith toward God for our family, friends, and community. The level of difference and influence varies from person to person, but the value and worth of the difference and influence is the same to God.

John 3:16 (NKJV) says, "For God so loved the world that He gave His only begotten Son, that whoever believes in Him should not perish but have everlasting life."

God loves us so much He sent His son to die for our sins so we may have confidence to enter His presence and seek His will for our lives. Jesus gave Himself for us because He knew how much His Father (who is also our Father) desired to be with us, so we may have wisdom, guidance, strength, and most of all, love for God and each other. God did this for the person who may influence a family and also for the person who may influence a country. The value and worth to God are the same; therefore, we must never look at what the believer next to us is doing and say, "I want to do that too," but rather we should always ask God, "What is my role in this world?"

A Prayer for the Called:

Matthew 14:25-33 (NKJV)

"Now in the fourth watch of the night Jesus went to them, walking on the sea. And when the disciples saw Him walking on the sea, they were troubled, saying, 'It is a ghost!' And they cried out for fear. But immediately Jesus spoke to them, saying, 'Be of good cheer! It is I; do not be afraid.' And Peter answered Him and said, "'Lord if it is You, command me to come to You on the water.' So, He said, 'Come.'

And when Peter had come down out of the boat, he walked on the water to go to Jesus. But when he saw that the wind was boisterous, he was afraid; and beginning to sink he cried out, saying, 'Lord, save me!' And immediately Jesus stretched out His hand and caught him, and said to him, 'O you of little faith, why did you doubt?' And when they got into the boat, the wind ceased. Then those who were in the boat came and worshiped Him, saying, 'Truly You are the Son of God.'"

Thank you, Father, for not leaving us where we are but coming down through Jesus to lift us up to Your presence. Thank you for faith, and may our faith be increased as the calls and challenges of life are revealed. May we have the courage of Peter to respond to Your call in faith and be willing to rise up from the position of spectator to participant believing that You have called us and will lead us through to finish what You have started. May our focus be on Your presence with us and help our faith triumph over our fears so we may continue to move forward. Thank you for lifting us up above our circumstances so we too may "walk on water" knowing You have every detail figured out and have our best interest in Your heart. May we call out to You when we feel like our faith falls short knowing You will respond. Jesus, You are the Son of God and we trust in You. Amen.

"Now the Lord spoke to Paul in the night by a vision, 'Do not be afraid, but speak, and do not keep silent; for I am with you, and no one will attack you to hurt you; for I have many people in the city.'"
– Acts 18:9-10 (AMP)

Part 2 - The Sharing

Yvette:

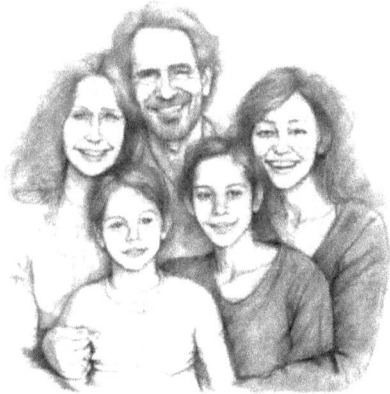

After the realization that Jake would one day need a kidney transplant, there was a lengthy period of uncertainty. Waiting can be so hard, especially when you don't know the when of the event that you know is going to have to take place one day. The diagnosis can change your perspective on life as my husband said. It made him realize that life is fragile, and Lori said it made her realize that life is not to be taken for granted and that she must learn to deal with the inevitable; she loves more than ever.

Our family continued the path before us; my husband, daughter, and I went to our jobs each day, and our sons went to school, played sports, and continued doing the things teenage boys do with their family and friends. We attended church, like always, and we participated in the home Bible studies, like always before. At times we could even almost forget that this needed transplant was around the corner. Jake handled it all so well. He remained happy and continued doing all the things he enjoyed in life as much as he could. His attitude was always amazing to me. He would say, "We will do what we have to do when the time comes." He was a fitting example to the rest of us to stay positive, to love and support each other, and to keep our faith strong, knowing God was in control.

You learn that in your weakness and feeling of helplessness you really need to share your concerns and allow others to be there for you, to support you, to pray for you, and to trust in the Lord. When we are facing something that is uncertain, scary, and even seemingly unfair, we tend to keep things to ourselves. Why? We feel that we do not want to burden others with our problems. Everyone has things going on in his/her life. We don't want to seem weak and that we are not able to handle something that has happened within our family that others may have experienced too. And yes, sometimes we even feel embarrassed, like we have done something wrong that has caused a problem we are facing. How wrong are we when we think this way? We are not being faithful to what God wants for us when we do this.

All throughout the Bible, there are over one hundred verses, in the Old and New Testaments, teaching us about how we are to share with and encourage each other. There is rejoicing because of encouragement. When we comfort and encourage each other, we are obeying God. As 2 Corinthians 1:3-4 (NIV) says, "Praise be to the God and Father of our Lord Jesus Christ, the Father of compassion and the God of all comfort, who comforts us in all our troubles, so that we may be able to comfort those who are in any trouble, with the comfort with which we ourselves receive from God." We are pleasing God when we put His teaching into practice by being there for others, just as Christ is there for us.

Being with our family, church family, and friends is so important for us and helps us to be encouraged and have hope for the future. Having support and Christian fellowship is life changing, not only in daily life, but most certainly in times when we are weak and facing challenging circumstances. Because we are human, we will definitely have our weak moments during difficult times.

When we went to his doctors' appointments for the needed checkups to test his glomerular filtration rate (GFR) and creatinine levels, the reality of all that was ahead for him would come back and cause fear and doubt in us each time. Being with others and talking and praying together would help us to have renewed strength and faith and remind us that because of these checkups, the doctors had the ability to know when time was getting closer. We were reminded that God was in control, and we had much to be thankful for even in these uncertain circumstances we were facing.

God never intended for us to be alone in our good or bad times. Fellowship with others is a blessing especially when we are facing an unknown; when we are scared and unsure which way to turn; and when we don't have all the answers for why certain things happen to us and our family. If we were alone in these times, without anyone to talk to or share with, we would become even more sad, worried, depressed, and even angry. How awful it would be if we did not have Christ in our lives and have other believers who we could come together with who could encourage us in prayer and thanksgiving and help us to keep our faith strong and remind us that God is always with us.

In Galatians 6:2 (NIV), God calls on us to "Carry each other's burdens, and in this way, you will fulfill the law of Christ." Fellowship builds friendships, unity, and faith in God. In our weakness, it helps us become stronger. By following God's Word in this verse, we are helping those in need by being kind, showing mercy, being sympathetic, and praying for them. Seeking help and sharing our concerns, our weakness, and our uncertainty through fellowship with others in Jesus' name makes us stronger, gives us a new perspective and a more positive outlook at what we are facing.

I'm reminded of 2 Corinthians 12:10 (NIV) that says, "That is why, for Christ's sake, I delight in weakness, in insults, in hardships, in persecutions, in difficulties. For when I am weak, then I am strong." This was Paul sharing after he was given some sort of affliction ("thorn" in his flesh, a "disease") as the Bible describes it. He pleaded with God three times to remove the affliction. God did not remove it. Paul then realized that when he was at his lowest, beaten down, and in pain, he then could feel God's power and presence the most.

Paul was declaring that whatever we face in our lives, whatever weakness we need help with—whether physical, mentally, emotionally, or spiritually—the grace of God, which is freely given to us by putting our faith (believing) in Jesus Christ, is always sufficient (adequate or enough) for our needs in this life and in the life to come. God's unchanging character gives us a firm foundation during our uncertainties. Trust in Him, talk with Him, and be obedient to His Word.

> *"When the righteous cry for help, the Lord hears and delivers them out of all their troubles."*
> – **Psalm 34:17** (ESV)

George:

Random connections have happened before. It happened in a Boston area Target parking lot in January 2022. A woman saw a sticker on a car for a person in need of a donation for a kidney and ended up talking to the patient herself. She was a match to donate and followed through with the surgery. These kinds of stories reinforce my belief that we are here to make a positive difference in each other's lives, but we have to be willing to act upon the prompts and engage with each other. This doesn't mean every prompt may end up as a glorious story to tell, but it does mean we will learn to follow through and trust that our lives are meant to be more than just lived for ourselves. This conviction carried me through the doubts I had about moving forward with testing. If I weren't a match, then I knew it was not to be, and I would have peace knowing I did what I could to help.

My blood samples were taken within a few days of the call and were sent to MUSC. I waited with great anticipation. I don't like to wait, and I don't know many people who do. In fact, I don't believe I know anyone who can say, "I like to wait." Thoughts of *what if* and *why me* come to mind while waiting, and I have learned to rejoice in these thoughts. *What if yes? Then praise God for matching me with this person! What if no? Then praise God for having something greater in mind! Why me? Then praise God for choosing me!* I don't say, Why me? with a downcast attitude. I say it with excitement and wonder. This can be hard to understand without a foundation of faith in God. Jesus teaches us all things are possible with God in Matthew chapter 19. This teaching comes to light when Jesus explains to His disciples how hard it is for the rich to enter the kingdom of heaven. The disciples thought the wealthy were blessed and, therefore, destined to heaven, but Jesus teaches that may not be the case. Material fortune does not always indicate God ordained spiritual blessing. Therefore, the disciples ask, "Who then can be saved?" Jesus replies in Matthew 19:27 saying, "With men this is impossible, but with God all things are possible"

(NKJV). All things are possible with God, and we can't do anything to build ourselves up to His presence. We need the grace of God through Jesus Christ, and by receiving His grace, we acknowledge a trust in God and His ability to bring us through the challenges of life. This truth can be hard to fathom, but we need to understand how everything, and I mean EVERYTHING in this world and in the heavens, is under God's sovereign control and available for His use to bring about His will.

An example of God's sovereignty from Scripture comes from how God brought Mary and Joseph to Bethlehem. The Messiah (Jesus Christ) was prophesied to be born in Bethlehem in the writings of the prophet Micah. Micah 5:2 (NJKV) says,

> *"But you, Bethlehem Ephrathah,*
> *Though you are little among the thousands of Judah,*
> *Yet out of you shall come forth to Me*
> *The One to be Ruler in Israel,*
> *Whose goings forth are from of old,*
> *From everlasting."*

Not long before Jesus was to be born, Mary and Joseph were living in Nazareth. This was far from Bethlehem in an area known as Galilee. From the human perspective, it may have seemed like this prophecy wasn't going to be fulfilled, or Mary wasn't going to truly give birth to the Messiah. But an angel told Mary that, "The Holy One who is to be born will be called the Son of God" in Luke 1:35 (NKJV). What I love the most are the last words the angel spoke to Mary in Luke 1:37: "For with God nothing will be impossible." Mary responds to the angel saying, "Let it be to me according to your word," in Luke 1:38. Mary had faith to believe because she believed God was speaking through the angel, but she still may have had doubts waiting in Nazareth as her due date approached. She also didn't do anything to prompt a move to Bethlehem and may not have even known about Micah's prophecy to begin with, but she trusted God.

God knows His plans and will complete what He says He will do because His word never returns void; in fact, another translation of Luke 1:37 says, "For the word of God will never fail" (NLT). God moved Mary and Joseph to Bethlehem using a census. In those days, people would return to their hometowns to register for a census, meaning Mary and Joseph would have to travel from Nazareth to Bethlehem! Scripture says,

> *"Joseph also went up from Galilee, out of the city of Nazareth,*
> *into Judea, to the city of David, which is called Bethlehem,*
> *because he was of the house and lineage of David, to be registered*
> *with Mary, his betrothed wife, who was this child. So it was*
> *that while they were there, the days were completed for her to be*
> *delivered. And she brought forth her firstborn Son, and wrapped*
> *Him in swaddling cloths, and laid Him in a manger, because*
> *there was no room for them in the inn."*
> **– Luke 2:4-7 (NKJV)**

May your faith be encouraged through this example of God's ability to use all things to bring His heavenly plans into our earthly existence. The fulfillment of Micah 5:2 didn't come through a great spiritual revelation. Instead the fulfillment came from obedience to an ordinary requirement of life during the ancient Roman Empire.

Don't overlook the simplicities of life and dismiss them as invaluable to God. I didn't know where my blood sample would lead, but I did know it was a step in the direction of compassion. I wanted to help and at least investigate the possibility of being a match for this person in need. God took the burden of worrying about all the details ahead because I knew I could trust Him because of His faithfulness to His Word and also from past experiences in my life. In other words, I believed that if this weren't meant to be, then it would not happen—and if it were meant to be, then all the details were already worked out.

I really wanted to be a match for this person because I love a great God story and was hopeful it would inspire others to trust God through Jesus. Nevertheless, I had to release my desire to the plans and purposes of God. I encourage you to continue to act upon the prompts for compassion and mercy. Embrace them out of love for God and desire for more of the world to experience His goodness. Move forward in faith knowing God's plans are far greater than what we can think or imagine and be bold to release all areas of your life for use by God. By God's grace, I took a step of faith the day I gave blood for testing by MUSC. I had no idea how great the change that first step would bring in my life and in the lives of many others.

A Prayer for the Sharing:

Luke 10:1-20 (NKJV)

I pray this passage of Scripture brings you joy as you read and reflect upon what God reveals. Luke 10 begins with Jesus sending seventy believers out into the surrounding region to preach the good news of the kingdom of God coming near.

Jesus says in Luke 10:8-9, "Whatever city you enter, and they receive you, eat such things as are set before you. And heal the sick there, and say to them, 'The kingdom of God has come near to you.'" Jesus also warns them about those who will not receive them and instructs them to "wipe the dust of their city off," but still leave with saying, "The kingdom of God has come near to you." Jesus also instructs them to travel without money, knapsack, or sandals in verse 4. He declares them to be like lambs among wolves in verse 3!

I don't know about you, but the declaration of being like a lamb among wolves does not give me great confidence. Traveling without money, a knapsack, or extra shoes doesn't seem wise either. In fact, it doesn't make sense going against worldly wisdom. Jesus was demanding the believers move in faith according to His Word. What happens? The believers go out two by two and return in Luke 10:17, "Then the seventy returned with joy, saying, 'Lord even the demons are subject to us in Your name.'"

Did the seventy return discouraged or disappointed? No, they returned with joy meaning with gladness, rejoicing, or bliss! Jesus continues to say the authority He has given them over all the power of the enemy but points out their true joy should come from the reality of their names being written in heaven: Luke 10:20, "Nevertheless do not rejoice in this, that the spirits are subject to you, but rather rejoice because your names are written in heaven."

Father God, may Your truth of writing our names in heaven through faith in Jesus be our source of joy! You have revealed Yourself as our Father, and we are Your children. Thank you for sending us out into the world as vessels of Your love, compassion, and mercy. May we be bold to proclaim the love You have for others through Jesus not only in word but through action as well. Show us where You desire us to reveal your love, and may we move forward in faith knowing Your work brings joy, gladness, rejoicing, and bliss! Thank you for working out the details and comforting us along the way. May we not fear where You send us, but trust You are not a God of disappointment, but a God of deliverance. In Jesus' name, Amen.

> *"These things I have spoken to you, that in Me you may have peace. In the world you will have tribulation; but be of good cheer, I have overcome the world."*
> **– John 16:33 (AMP)**

Part 3 - The Testing

Yvette:

I was ready to be tested as soon as I knew that Jake would need a kidney, but of course, testing for me would wait until his kidneys showed that signs of failing were closer. Time would only tell when that would be. I did, however, tell the doctors that when it was time, I wanted to be the one to donate if I were a good match. I was not familiar with any of the testing processes at all. I had not known anyone before that needed a kidney transplant or any other transplant of any kind, but I did know that my son would need one, and I had no doubt at all that I would be the first to be tested to see if I could do this for him. I began to read so many wonderful stories of others donating to family and even strangers; it filled my heart with joy thinking I could do this too, especially for my own son.

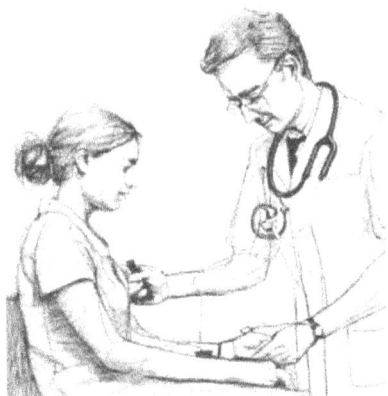

1 John 5:14 (NKJV) says, "This is the confidence we have in approaching God: that if we ask anything according to his will, He hears us." This was my faith prayer with submission. I did not know the outcome, but I did know that God could certainly make it happen if it were His will to do so.

By studying the Word of God, believing it, repenting of my sins, and confessing my belief in Jesus Christ by being baptized, I had this confidence and assurance that He does hear my every prayer. He hears me having conversations with Him, praising Him, glorifying His name, giving thanks, sharing my thoughts and concerns, and confiding in Him everything I need to talk about.

I told all my family and friends that I would be the donor for Jake, no questions asked. I would be the first to be tested, and I asked them for their prayers for the outcome to prove for me to be a good match to be able do this.

Gary knew that I wanted to be the donor, and nothing he could say would ever, ever change my mind. Lori was not surprised one bit that I wanted to be the donor, except she did wonder why I chose to do that before she or Jason because they were younger, but when I explained that Jake would probably need another kidney in the future, she then saw clearly why I wanted to do this first. She was worried about me but shared that I was one tough lady, and she would be there to help me recover and comfort me. What more could I want? Jason shared when asked what he thought about his mom donating a kidney to Jake. "I think my mom was born to do that. She would lay down her life for us all, and we've known that since we were very young. She instilled that in us."

During the waiting time, God allowed Jake to get through high school and graduate with his brother, Jason. He was also able to be a groomsman for his sister Lori at her wedding before it was time for the transplant. He had faced some sickness along the way but nothing that kept him down for long. He was living his life to the fullest as much as he could. He had peace and trust in God that what needed to be done would be at the right time.

God always has our back and desires to bless us. Along with being able to graduate with his brother and be in his sister's wedding, we were also able to take Jake and Jason to the World Cup Soccer Games that year in Florida after their graduation with the tickets we had surprised them with as a graduation present. All the things we had hoped and prayed to accomplish before the transplant was granted. The very next checkup showed that the time for a transplant had come. God's timing is always perfect.

The appointments were scheduled for me to be tested right away. We were anxious for things to be done quickly so if I were not a good match, another family member could be tested right away. I still felt confident that I would be a match. I wanted to be first so Gary, my husband, could continue to work and provide for us, and when Jake needed another kidney, his sister or brother could be used and hopefully last longer than this first one I hoped to be giving him. The scheduling was so efficient at Charlotte Medical Center, and the process went smoothly. Just like with George's experience at MUSC, the staff was so caring, making me feel like I was one of the most special people in the world during the entire process. The team of transplant doctors were excellent, as were the medical technicians and the nursing staff. They were always there to answer questions, be helpful, and were efficient in every way. All tests were performed promptly so results could be studied as soon as possible. The disease inside Jake was working extremely fast now.

The results were studied, and I was thrilled to hear I would be a good match and could be the donor. God had answered our prayers with a perfect chain of events taking place. As soon as the results were reviewed by the team, it was time for the surgery to be scheduled to take place. The wonderful staff and the transplant team were making everything happen quickly. It was all like perfect clockwork and like we, alone, were their top priority; that was how they made us feel!

Oh, how much better off we were instead of wondering and worrying about things to come. Instead, we memorized and took to heart the verse of Proverbs 16:9, "In their hearts humans plan their course, but the Lord establishes their steps" (NIV). Amen!

God is all knowing. His plans for us always exceed any expectations that we could ever hope for or imagine when we trust in Him. Trust in Him in all things. He hears us; He knows what we will need and when we will need it.

"'For I know the plans I have for you,' declares the Lord,
'plans to prosper you and not to harm you, plans to give
you hope and a future. Then you will call on me and come
and pray to me, and I will listen to you.'"
– Jeremiah 29:11 (NIV)

During the time the above verse was written in the Bible, Babylonia became an immensely powerful city. The prophet, Jeremiah, was told to warn the Jews about the crime and destruction that was going to happen to destroy Jerusalem. Many were following false prophets and were living in sin and did not listen to Jeremiah's warning to repent and escape ruin. The people did not obey God's word, and Babylon captured Jerusalem twice—once in 605 BC and again in 598 BC. After being captured the second time, the remaining Jews were forced into exile to Babylon for seventy years. Even in their exile, which the Lord allowed because of their disobedience to Him, He was still watching over them. He told them to build houses there, have families, and increase so that they would not diminish and to seek the peace for the city of Babylon, where He caused them to be carried away to, and pray to the Lord for it; for in its peace, they would also have peace.

Even though they did not listen to Jeremiah, the prophet of truth, the Lord told them not to listen to false prophets and promised them that after the seventy years in Babylon, He would visit them, perform His Good Word toward them, and allow them to return to their home, Jerusalem, and rebuild the temple there. As the verse above says, His plans for them were a good life, not a life in exile, but He wanted them to diligently seek Him, love Him, and fulfill His purpose for their lives.

This is the same He wants for us and from us today. He knows the plans He has for us, but they can only be discovered when we obey Him. He will hear our prayers when we do this and fulfill His good plans for us.

In times of needing a kidney, a heart, a liver, or in any medical situation when we seek God's help, first accept Jesus, believe in Him, and trust and obey God's Word. This will give you confidence in the power of your prayers, and you can have rest knowing God will answer them according to His will.

Being tested to be a living donor is not a challenging thing to go through. You are well taken care of throughout the entire process and show love for others by being willing to help in their time of need. You are serving as God asks of us; not just to love ourselves, but to love others also.

Being an organ donor is one of the best feelings you will ever have, knowing you were able to be a Life Saver for another person. The love and appreciation that you will receive in return will change your life.

Please start with a few blood tests to see if you can be a donor. If God calls you to consider this, please do not ignore His guiding you there to serve in that way. Be in prayer about it and open to what He has planned for you and for the recipient.

There is a beautiful song that comes to mind when I think about being willing to serve in this way. The song, "Here I Am, Lord," written by Dan Schutte in 1979 when he was 31-years-old and studying theology at the Jesuit School of Theology at Berkeley. The lyrics were inspired by the Bible verses Isaiah 6:8 and 1 Samuel 3 as his song is a testament to Schutte's Godly devotion, emphasizing a willingness to act in accordance with the will of the Lord.

The chorus of the song expresses praise and worship and thanks for the Lord's amazing involvement in our lives. The words are written as:

"Here I am, Lord. Is it I, Lord?
I have heard You calling in the night.
I will go, Lord if You lead me
I will hold Your people in my heart."

With thoughtful prayer, be willing to say, "Here I am, Lord" if you are called to be a donor. Share the love of God and love for God's people, our brothers and sisters in Christ.

Bobbie:

My son proceeded to undergo the extensive testing required for prospective living kidney donors. From my understanding, the testing involved spending two days in Charleston with one day being the tests themselves and the other day being discussions with doctors. For a reason I don't remember now, I couldn't go with him.

I may have had more questions to ask the doctors than he did, so I did my best to relay them through him. I want my children to be healthy, but a part of me hoped there would be some finding through the testing that would disqualify my son from becoming a donor. The idea of my son becoming a living donor did not sit well with me. I did not like the idea and hoped this idea would pass; but I also thought the testing wasn't a commitment to donate and only a next step in the pursuit of more information.

My son proceeded to spend the two days in Charleston, and all his travel expenses were covered through the National Living Donor Assistance Center. I thought MUSC did an excellent job of explaining all the resources available to potential living donors to help offset the cost of traveling for tests and doctor discussions. The hospital staff gave him a clear picture of what would happen the day of the testing and who he would be able to speak with the day of the test results and discussions.

I was confident in my son's ability to navigate the visit, but I still wanted to be there. A mother wants to be there for her children, especially when they are taking big risks or moving into a new adventure in life. Nevertheless, the timing just didn't work out, and I would have to wait for his report.

I am used to waiting for my son though. A few years before this living donor idea came to his mind, he was an avid runner and covered every distance from a 5k to the marathon. I would travel with him to many of the longer races, including a few trips to New York and Boston. If you have ever entertained a running friend or family member by traveling with them to a race, then you can understand the amount of waiting that takes place. There is a lot of excitement building up to the start, and then they're off! If it's a marathon, then my son wouldn't be returning for at least a little over three hours. His running time left me a lot of time to wait. I am used to it, but that doesn't make it easy or the most enjoyable. Of course, getting to see him cross the finish line of a race was very exciting, especially if it was a marathon.

In some ways, his testing was like a race. He would be off early in the morning, and I knew I may not hear from him until much later in the day. This new journey brought excitement to him, and I supported him and cheered him on much like I would on race day. Not long after he finished his time with the tests and doctors, he let me know all went well, but it would be a few weeks before a final decision would be made about the possibility of him becoming a living donor. Again, I continued to hope something would distract or take away this thought from my son. I continued to try and understand why he thought this was a good idea. I thought he should be thinking about what this may do to his future health and how this may take away from doing other activities he loves like running and exercising. Parents want to see their children grow up into the best versions of themselves, and up to this point, I remained unconvinced of this being the way.

George:

I believe I followed through with the call to compassion by submitting to blood tests to see if I were a match for the person in need of a kidney transplant. I waited with great anticipation for the results with the hope of being able to help. I have been blessed with a healthy body. I have had challenges, of course, including asthma as a child, but by God's grace, I have endured, thrived, and overcome. My asthma was so bad as a youth, I often had to have special breathing treatments in the middle of the night and carried a rescue inhaler wherever I went. Because of this, I often avoided sports or activities that required lots of physical activity for fear of an asthma attack. Looking back, I do believe I would have enjoyed being more involved in sports through high school, especially running, but I have peace knowing it wasn't the time. I am thankful for where I am today and what God has allowed me to do. My asthma has subsided for the most part, and my late-night breathing treatments are long gone. I became very interested in physical health after turning thirty and began to run. I liked the simplicity of running as exercise. No gym membership or expensive equipment were required, just a t-shirt, shorts, socks, and shoes. I ran out the front door through the neighborhood where I lived and just kept going.

I entered 5k races, which motivated me to run with purpose.

I wanted to see how fast I could go! I struggled in the races at first, but I endured and crossed the finish line. I did not envision this happening when I first began running, but thanks to the motivation of co-workers and my curiosity to see how far I could go, I eventually entered half and full marathons. The 5k (3.1 miles) distance was not enough to satisfy my desire for distance and challenge. Not only did I want to see how fast I could go, but now I wanted to see how far. I finished my first marathon distance race (26.2 miles) in 2011 and continued to look for more races to enter.

The marathon distance is like a jungle adventure. You have a map so the chances of getting lost are low, but you still don't know what will happen between the start and finish. A lot can change over the course of 26.2 miles, and this unknown experience and adventure excited me. I start a race with great expectation of running fast and finishing strong. Months of hard work go into serious marathon training, and as I moved on from my first marathon race in 2011, my training diversified and intensified. I watched what I ate more than ever and became vegetarian for a while. I became a lean running machine and even qualified and ran the Boston marathon in 2016. I enjoyed my ability to run the marathon distance and didn't pursue anything further. I believe in running practical distances, and anything over 26.2 miles doesn't make sense. I have no interest in being on a running course for twelve, eighteen, or twenty-four hours, but I do cheer on those who make that choice. All the running, cross training, and disciplined eating habits brought me to the best shape of my life.

Could it be that being blessed with health means that I should do something more with it than run races? As I reflected on my decision to have blood tests and what the results may bring, I thought, *What if I have been blessed with a healthy body, so I can help someone else who is less fortunate?* Yes, I did the work to get healthy (and it was a lot of work) but the ability to do so was given to me. For whatever reason I recognize, not everyone is able or gifted with the desire to run a marathon or run at all. We all have different gifts, and I believe the blessings of those gifts are not meant to be limited to ourselves, family, or friends. We exist to help each other regardless of race, color, or creed, and the diversity of gifts and abilities we all have testifies to this truth. Like an orchestra, when musicians play their parts with their specific instrument in tune, the results are a harmonious beautiful sound. But if the musicians miss their part or the instruments are not in tune, then the results will not be music to the audiences' ears. Humanity can accomplish great things and live in peace, but we all have to do our part and work together recognizing we are here to help each other without limitation. To the one who is blessed with finances, help those who have less. To the one who is blessed with wisdom, may that wisdom be shared. And to the one who is blessed with health, may that health be used to bring healing to someone else. Sharing health could be the sharing of experience or knowledge or thanks to medical advancement, sharing a kidney.

Not long after the blood tests, I received a call from a living donor transplant team member saying I wasn't a match. Part of me was disappointed, but there was also some relief. This news also left me with a question, What do I do now? My eyes had been opened to a need and to the possibility of being able to help by becoming a living kidney donor. Before my phone call to MUSC on that day in Florence, SC, I had the limited thinking that only family members could donate organs to one another. I really believed that there had to be that close of a genetic connection for the possibility to become reality. The great people on the MUSC transplant team educated me. They also asked me if I was interested in becoming a living kidney donor for someone else. There would be a significant amount of testing involved meaning I would have to spend two nights in Charleston, SC, to complete it all. Again, thoughts of excitement and wonder came into my head, and I said, "Let's go!"

The seed had been planted in my mind about the possibility of becoming a living kidney donor. I shared this thought with family, friends, and co-workers and received a well-blended mix of responses. Some were excited, some were curious, some flat out said no, and my family especially expressed concern. The most common question people would ask of me was, "What if?" What if I needed my other kidney later in life? What if someone in my family needed a kidney? What if a close friend needed one? What if I needed to have two because one began to fail? No doubt these are all valid responses and did prompt me to give careful consideration to pursuing the living donation process, but most questions were settled by, "Let me pursue the testing, and we will go from there." I mean after all, "What if I don't get approved to donate or the tests find my kidneys need medical attention?" Those around me were comforted by this logic, and I felt confident moving forward and made a commitment to my assigned test days.

I covered this entire process with prayer and asked others to join me too. My church family, my Bible study group, and others committed to pray for wisdom and guidance. Now I saw a great need for living kidney donors. My workplace received an email from a brother who wanted to help his sister receive a kidney. I received Val-Pak advertisements in the mail of people in need of kidney transplants. I also met a pastor who was on the receiving end of a living donor, and he shared his story with me too. The testing days couldn't come soon enough!

Testing time arrived and the MUSC staff is serious when they say, "Pack a lunch." I can testify to this truth and back it up by saying, "Unless you want your early morning fast for blood work to continue through the entire day, you better pack a lunch." I awoke early as normal for a gathering with friends over the phone to pray and seek God's guidance for the day. I enjoy starting my day in prayer to God and reading the Bible because this routine helps motivate my thoughts and actions toward heaven. It also reminds me that yesterday is gone, be thankful for today, and remember I am loved. I find early mornings to be a great time of inspiration and motivation, and I am thankful I got to share that early morning with so many people whom I love.

MUSC had a serious schedule outlined with most minutes of the day covered by blood work, ultrasounds, x-rays, and kidney scans. The staff was excellent and extremely helpful and also very efficient. I felt prepared for the day and was very thankful I packed a lunch. Because of a lot of moving around from one medical department to another, the day went by pretty quickly, and before I knew it, I was walking back to my hotel room for the evening. My thankful thoughts continued throughout the evening as I rejoiced in having a smooth day of testing. My thoughts also focused on, *What if I am approved to donate? The seed has been planted and sprouted but would it grow any further? Is it supposed to grow any further?* I wasn't sure, but I knew a path would be revealed, and I rested. We live in an amazing time when you consider organs from one human can be shared with another.

As a Christian, I believe one of the greatest calls in my life, and in the lives of all Christians, is to release your rights to results. Release your rights to God through the revelation of Jesus dying for you to bringing you into the presence of God. God did this out of love for His creation and the desire to not just be with one nation but with the entire world. John 3:16 (NKJV) says,

> *"For God so loved the world that He gave*
> *His only begotten son that whoever believes*
> *in Him will not perish but have eternal life."*

A key to receive this blessing from God is to humble ourselves before God. When we recognize we aren't meant to live our life alone spiritually and that God desires for us to be guided by Him, we release our rights of desire for our outcomes to God. In other words, we say, "God I am here for You and may You be glorified through my life." We don't have to work to receive God's love because John 3:16 shows us God loved us before we loved Him and through the release of our desires, we open the door to receive the fullness of blessing from God. This release does not mean missing out; rather it means a level up and a joining in the greatest call you can have upon your life. Not only will you have profound change in your life and affect the lives of those immediately around you, but you will also change the world by remaining in communion with God through Jesus Christ.

Jesus reveals the struggle of humanity to release all roles and outcomes into God's hands in the Garden of Gethsemane in the last hours of His life. Remember from the beginning of His arrival on earth and even before time began, Jesus knew God's plan. He knew the outcome of the cross, but He also knew He still had to go through the process. What did Jesus do in the garden? He prayed to God and asked His disciples to join Him in prayer. The synoptic gospels of Matthew, Mark, and Luke record this experience. I especially like Luke's record because it shows the agony and struggle Jesus faced in His humanity as His suffering and death drew near. Jesus' first words to His disciples in Luke 22:40 (NIV) were, ***"On reaching the place, he said to them, 'Pray that you may not enter into temptation.'"*** Those *what ifs* can be a distraction and doorway to temptation if we lose focus on our connection with God's plans and purposes. Jesus shows us prayer keeps us focused on God's plans. When we pray, God responds.

Luke 22:41-44 (NKJV) says,

> *"And He was withdrawn from them about a*
> *stone's throw, and He knelt down and prayed, saying,*
> *'Father, if it is Your will, take this cup away from Me;*
> *nevertheless not My will, but Yours, be done.' Then an*
> *angel appeared to Him from heaven, strengthening Him.*
> *And being in agony, He prayed more earnestly.*
> *Then His sweat became like great drops of*
> *blood falling down to the ground."*

The drops of blood in Luke's record reveal the deep struggle of Jesus' humanity to fully submit to the will of God, but what does Jesus say? "Not My will, but Yours be done," in Luke 22:42 (NKJV). Jesus knew the pain of the scourging and crucifixion would be great. He knew His physical body would suffer, and it would be as if God had forsaken Him leaving Him alone to die on a cross, but He found strength through prayer and knowing what was to come on the other side of the cross, so He endured. Jesus endured not by His own strength but through God's. Jesus didn't endure through His humanity, but He endured through the spiritual strength and guidance God gives His children when they ask for help. Jesus released His body to the will of God that evening in the garden because He knew the pain would ultimately be limited and the glory forever.

Now in no way am I comparing my experience of kidney donation to the level of Jesus on the cross, but I want to offer the mention of Scriptures as a lesson for us to have peace in releasing our physical bodies to the service of God. We can't have this release without the power of God in our lives. Our vision will remain limited, and we will ultimately choose to preserve ourselves. Jesus showed how real this struggle can be, and I pray you find comfort in knowing even the Son of God contended with the thought of self-preservation. Jesus contended and conquered the thought by releasing His rights to God through prayer and allowing His spiritual strength to surpass the nature of humanity. When we humble ourselves before God like Jesus and say, "Not my will, but Yours be done," we open the door and invite God to work through our lives. In other words, we are saying, "I trust in God to lead me into fulfilling His plans because they are so much better than mine, even if they mean facing trial and going through suffering. Because of Your unfailing love, I know the pain will be limited and the glory will last forever."

A Prayer for the Testing:

The apostle Paul writes about pressing toward the goal in his letter to the Philippians. He writes in Philippians 3:12-14 (NKJV), *"Not that I have already attained or am already perfected: but I press on, that I may lay hold of that for which Christ Jesus has also laid hold of me. Brethren, I do not count myself to have apprehended; but one thing I do, forgetting those things which are behind and reaching forward to those things which are ahead. I press toward the goal for the prize of the upward call of God in Christ Jesus."*

Paul expresses his humility before God and reveals his desire to continue to move forward with God by "forgetting those things which are behind and reaching forward to those things which are ahead." He releases the past and doesn't allow past mistakes or experiences to hold him back from pursuing the will of God for his life. He embraces the day and presses toward the goal God has for his life in Christ Jesus. I pray this continues to be our desire too.

Father God, help us to continually release our will to Yours. May we pause and consider what Your desires for our lives are on a daily basis and go after them with a fervor like Paul. May we too continue to press on and move forward with You as you lead us through our existence in this world knowing Your plans and purposes are far greater than what we can think or imagine. Help us to see beyond the immediate trial or suffering to see Your glory through it and Your strength to endure it. May we not be afraid to cry out to You just like Jesus did in the garden of Gethsemane and ask for help. May we involve others around us and find strength in prayer. May we not fall into temptation but be delivered from evil in Jesus' name. Amen.

"I would have lost heart, unless I believed that I would see the goodness of the Lord in the land of the living."
– Psalm 27:13 (NKJV)

Part 4 - The Waiting

Yvette:

Researchers really do not know exactly what causes this kidney disease, and the disease may have slowly been destroying Jake's kidneys for years and years without any symptoms present.. This left us feeling like we were not good parents for not realizing something was going on inside his seemingly healthy body.

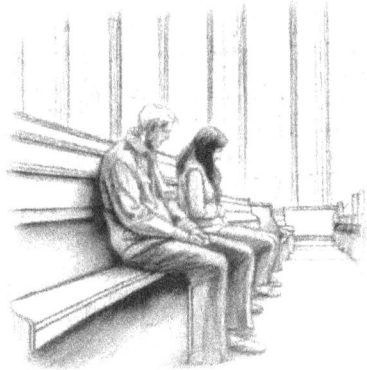

After more tests and a biopsy of his kidneys, the disease called IgA Nephropathy (Berger's Disease) was diagnosed. There is no cure for this disease. It is an autoimmune disease that attacks the kidneys and affects how blood is filtered in the blood vessels of the kidneys. The kidneys can begin to stop functioning and lead to kidney failure for some people, and others will not experience any complications at all. The disease may even go into remission on its own. However, some people develop more complications as the condition progresses.

Our son was one of those people who would have complications including high blood pressure, high cholesterol, acute kidney failure, possible heart problems, and end-stage renal disease, meaning he would need a kidney transplant one day.

We were devastated for him. It did not seem real; he had always been so healthy. Thank God for the doctor who gave him a thorough physical and discovered this when he did.

After learning more about this disease, we found there could be both genetic and environmental components that cause it. A person can be born with a predisposition for the disease. Some type of trigger (an exposure to something or an infection) can occur and make the disease progress. If there isn't a trigger, there may never be a problem. We tried to relive the years thinking if there was something we missed along the way. We did recall that he had been bitten once in the foot by an insect we never found, and his foot had swollen. Could this have been the trigger? We would not know for sure, but it would be a life-long disease that he would have to learn to live with.

One of the hard parts was that lots of waiting would be involved. There was no way to know when the transplant would be needed. Only Jake's body and the continued check-ups would determine the time.

That was a hard pill to swallow at times. Most of us are impatient just having to wait for a minute, let alone wait indefinitely. There are many things we wait for—some are good things that we wait for: the birth of a baby, the return of someone coming home that has been gone for a long time, and others we do not particularly like to wait for at times like dinner to be cooked, clothes to dry, etc. Then, of course, there are things we think of as unbearable and wonder how we will ever get through the waiting. This is when, even though we don't understand why things like this must happen to our loved ones, we must stop, remember who is in control, and hand over our burdens, our hurt, and yes, even our anger to our Heavenly Father about what is happening. He is always with us and keeps us as if in the palm of His hand, when we believe, trust, and obey His Word.

When you know something must happen, but you don't know when, the waiting seems so hard. Yes, we usually have our family and our friends to talk to and listen to us about our concerns. That certainly helps, but unless we have faith and the assurance from our Heavenly Father that we have the Holy Spirit within us, comforting us, and showing us the way to be patient and let God's will be done, it would be almost unbearable.

"Our family has always been close; that helped us handle this," said Lori. This was Lori's answer when she was asked if it did bring us closer. "We were on a mission to get this need handled and focus on the facts and what had to be done. We band together whenever one needs the other, no questions asked! I can assure you, you cannot break our bond no matter what. We all have faith that God is in control, and our strength comes from Him."

Think of storms. Storms can come out of nowhere, and they can come quickly without warning. They can be mild storms, or they can become megastores. Storms can also have significant impacts on those involved in the storm. They can rain on the righteous or the unrighteous; there is no picking or choosing who the storms will affect. BUT remember that the Lord can calm the storms. Our job through the storms of life is to be willing to gain spiritual knowledge by pursuing the truth and giving our lives to Jesus and rejoice even in the challenging times. The trials in life are part of our journey. Romans 5:1-5 (NIV) teaches us about peace and hope.

> *"Therefore, since we have been justified through faith, we have a peace with God through our Lord Jesus Christ, through whom we have gained access by faith into this grace in which we now stand. And we boast in the hope of the glory of God. Not only that, but we also boast about our sufferings, knowing that suffering produces endurance, endurance produces character, and character produces hope. Now this hope does not disappoint us, because God's love has been poured out into our hearts by the Holy Spirit, who has been given to us."*

> *"Rejoice in hope, be patient in tribulation, be constant in prayer."*
> **– Romans 12:12 (NIV)**

Yes, the waiting and wondering can seem endless and feel like we will never have the answers we are seeking, but that is when we really need to stop and think about the waiting and wondering that Jesus endured when He was on His way to the cross so we could be forgiven for our sins and be able to pray to God through Jesus Christ. We must give thanks and praise His name for His love for us and have blessed assurance that He is with us every step of our journey in this life if we have accepted Him as our Lord and Savior. I recall hearing a friend talking about how people are so impatient even in church at times. A particular person in church seemed to take it upon himself/herself to think for the whole congregation, always questioning the pastor about how much time was being taken for certain parts of the service and even complaining about how long the Christmas services were lasting.

I was shocked to hear that they had suggested the Christmas Eve service should not be over a certain amount of time because "People really don't want to be here on Christmas Eve; they want to get home to be with family and open a Christmas Eve gift instead of sitting in church for a long time," as they put it! WOW!

My friend put it in perspective when she remembered about the waiting time of Jesus as He was waiting to be hung on the cross. His waiting involved being mocked, beaten, tortured, and having to carry his own cross to the place He would be crucified, followed by more waiting until His actual death.

How could people at church complain about the time they had to be at church longer than they wanted to be before they could go home and do what they really wanted to be doing! Could they not even give an hour praising God and being thankful for all that Jesus endured for each of us?

> *"But as for me, I will look to the Lord; I will wait for the*
> *God of my salvation; My God will hear me."*
> **– Micah 7:7 (NIV)**

Turn your waiting and wondering time into time spent with your Heavenly Father filled with praise and thanksgiving because of the goodness of God.

George:

Most of us do a lot of waiting in life. Waiting in lines, traffic, seeing a doctor, or picking up our child from school are just a few examples. Amusement parks create elaborate immersive waiting areas before rides. Restaurants provide places to sit while waiting for a table, and medical offices have rooms dedicated to waiting. No matter who you are, at some point in your life, you are going to have to wait. Even the rich and famous have to wait. The question is not if you have to wait, but **when you have to wait, how well do you wait?** In the past, I haven't waited well. My patience would wear out, and I would give in to frustration and discontent, attempting to force a solution instead of relaxing and releasing the outcome to God. This does not mean disengagement from seeking solutions or being involved in the outcome of a trial of time, but it does mean peace and patience through the process. Be prepared to wait in your life, and be prepared to wait longer than expected. If you prepare for it, then you can bear it and experience joy through the process.

The times of waiting can be the greatest challenges of our faith. I waited eighteen months between being approved to donate a kidney and the donation operation itself. I battled thoughts of insignificance, wrongdoing, and doubt. At times I was tempted to call MUSC and go back on my willingness to donate. I thought if God was leading me to this, then the need must be immediate. I did not think I would be waiting eighteen months for the operation. I wondered if maybe the need wasn't as great as advertised. I thought, *Maybe I am not supposed to make this decision.* I doubted God led me into the opportunity. The truth is becoming a living organ donor is a complicated process, and lots of boxes have to be checked, and everything has to be in perfect order before a transplant can proceed. This takes time.

My victory against those thoughts always came back to the truth of my relationship with God through Jesus Christ. Through Jesus, God reveals Himself as a good Father who wants to be in relationship with His children. Because He is a good Father, He sometimes has to delay or restrain certain events from our lives because He knows the time isn't right. We want it now, but our Father in heaven says no or not yet. Trusting in God and His ways, processes, and timing will give you strength and hope through a trial of time. His plans are the best.

Don't give up! I am always encouraged by the many people in the Bible who waited well. They kept their *antennas* up for God and continued to live their lives for God while waiting on God. They didn't feel sorry for themselves and beat themselves up thinking they had failed. They didn't give in to thoughts of doubt or despair. They continued to look up and live on through their hope that the day would come when they would see the goodness of God in the land of the living! John the Baptist's parents are great examples of waiting well. Luke chapter 1 tells us Zacharias and Elizabeth were advanced in age and had never had children.

Luke 1:6-7 (NKJV) says, "And they were both righteous before God, walking in all the commandments and ordinances of the Lord blameless. But they had no child, because Elizabeth was barren, and they were both well advanced in years." Understand what these verses say to us today: Living for God and obeying God does not mean immediate response from God. I do not doubt for a moment that Zacharias and Elizabeth battled thoughts that were against God. I am sure they heard lies in their head trying to get them to give up on God and walk away from serving Him because it's not worth it. They didn't give in and waited well. Zacharias continued to serve God in the temple as he was assigned, and Elizabeth remained faithful to her part as well. They encouraged each other and held onto their belief in a God who loves them. They built their lives on the foundation of this truth.

If your faith is wavering through this time of trial, Luke 1:13-17 (NKJV) should give you great encouragement. Zacharias is called to burn incense in the temple of the Lord. This can only be done once in a priest's career and Zacharias had been called. One of perhaps eighteen thousand priests at the time, Zacharias had been chosen. Zacharias proceeds with his calling and enters the temple of the Lord to burn the incense. While inside he encounters an angel of the Lord. Luke 1:13-17 (NKJV) says,

"But the angel said to him, 'Do not be afraid,
Zacharias, for your prayer is heard; and your
wife Elizabeth will bear you a son, and you shall
call his name John. And you will have joy
and gladness, and many will rejoice at

his birth. For he will be great in the sight
of the Lord and shall drink neither wine
nor strong drink. He will also be filled with
the Holy Spirit even from his mothers' womb.
And he will turn many of the children of
Israel to the Lord their God. He will also go
before Him in the spirit and power of Elijah,
to turn the hearts of the fathers to the children,
and the disobedient to the wisdom of the just,
to make ready a people prepared for the Lord."'

In other words, Zacharias and Elizabeth will not only be blessed with a child, but they will also be blessed with a child who will be filled with the Holy Spirit and will help lead the children of Israel back to the Lord their God through Jesus.

All of this begins with Luke 1:13 (NKJV) as the angel says, "For your prayer has been heard." Zacharias and Elizabeth had been praying for a child. They may have been praying specifically for a son. The point is they were asking God through prayer and God reminds Zacharias through the angel that He heard the prayer. God hears your prayers too, and the example of Zacharias and Elizabeth is a great lead to follow. They prayed and they waited. They asked God and they continued to serve God while they waited on God. They didn't give up, and the day came when God did what only He could do. Advanced in age and beyond the normal expectation of childbearing years, God brought John the Baptist through Elizabeth. The gifts of God are greater than we can think or imagine. Ephesians 3:20-21 (NKJV) says,

"Now to Him who is able to do exceedingly abundantly
above all that we ask or think, according to the power
that works in us, to Him be glory in the church by
Christ Jesus to all generations forever and ever, Amen."

You may be waiting to receive an organ, or you may be waiting to donate an organ, and God knows you are waiting. Remember, God's plans, answers, and timing are not below what you ask or think but exceedingly abundantly above! The moments of deliverance are greater, so don't give up and continue to wait with great expectation.

A Prayer for the Waiting:

Joshua 1:8 (NKJV) says, "Keep this Book of the Law (Book of the Torah) always on your lips; meditate on it day and night, so that you may be careful to do everything written in it. Then you will be prosperous and successful." In other words, God says, "Remain in My presence; follow Me; trust Me." He asks, "Have I not revealed Myself to you?" Our Father in Heaven loves us as His children and the way through the waiting is to remain in His presence.

Joshua 1:9 (NKJV) says, "Have I not commanded you? Be strong and courageous. Do not be afraid; do not be discouraged, for the LORD your God will be with you wherever you go." Our call is to be strong and courageous like Joshua. Our call is to be patient and faithful while we wait on God's timing. We must never give up because He has given us His promise to be with us wherever we go. God is with you in the waiting. He is with you in the heartache. He is with you in the challenge. And He will lead you through to a deliverance that is greater, more profound, and life changing than you can even imagine. Glorify God with your life in all seasons and know that the season of waiting won't last forever. Winter gives way to spring, spring to summer, and then the harvest is reaped. Your harvest is coming, but you must follow through with what Paul writes in 1 Corinthians 15:57-58 (NKJV), "But thanks be to God, who gives us the victory through our Lord Jesus Christ. Therefore, my beloved brethren, be steadfast, immovable, always abounding in the work of the Lord, knowing that your labor is not in vain in the Lord."

Father God, Your plans are perfect. May we stay steadfast in Your presence, trusting that what You have begun You will bring to a glorious completion. May the desires of our heart not be removal of the troubling circumstance or discomfort but rather a trust in Your path through the challenge. May we continue to live in hope and the blessed assurance of Your presence in the seasons of waiting. And when our time of waiting has ended, may we be strong and courageous like Joshua. May Your words be the center of our lives and may our voices glorify Your name for the deliverance. Your will be done in Jesus' name. Amen.

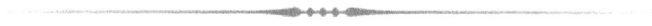

Part 5 - The Findings

Yvette:

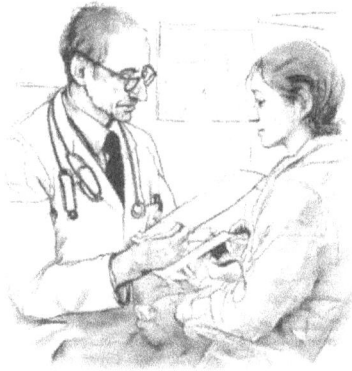

I suppose you could say I was a little full of myself when it came to the findings after all the tests were completed. I was just so sure that I was going to be the donor for Jake that I didn't give the proper thought and appreciation that I should have during it all. Thankfully, God had already set the path for this before I had so selfishly declared to everyone that I was going to be the donor to my son for this first kidney he needed. Yes, I was in constant prayer to my Heavenly Father that all would go well, but I was not giving Him the glory through my praying. I felt I was his mother, and as his mother, I would give him more life in this way than I could. I did not give any thought to the possibility that there could be some hidden problem or disease in my body that may have caused me not to be able to do this. I was in my forties, fit and healthy in my mind, so this was going to happen. I didn't stop to think about the fact that we thought Jake was fit and healthy with no problems, but then this not known disease had been working inside of him for years that changed everything for him. There easily could have been something, maybe even the same disease, working inside of me that we didn't know about since some people have the same disease, and it's never triggered to become a problem where a transplant is needed.

But God in his love, mercy, and grace (and probably shaking His head at me) was in control, and He had already had this path beautifully laid out for me to be the donor to my precious son. I was so very thankful and happy when I was called and told that I would in fact be able to do this. I did not have any hidden disease that would prevent me from being the living donor, and even though the surgery was more difficult in 1994 than it is today, I was in great health and would have no problems that were foreseen.

The nurses and doctors felt like family by this time, and I was so completely at peace with it all. I could not wait until the day it would all happen. I was more than ready to see Jake feel good again and to be able to continue his young life without having to worry about a disease that had gone unknown for so many years. Yes, we were told that he would one day need another transplant because the disease does continue to weaken and eventually destroy even the new kidney, but we had faith that it would be many, many years before that would be needed. So, with our faith in God and the knowledge that we had some of the top surgeons taking care of him, we chose to put it in God's hands and not live our days until then in worry and fear, but in celebration of each new day we were given to enjoy happiness and health in our lives.

We were blessed that Jake had living donors available to him, and I realize that not everyone in need of an organ transplant has this situation available to them. That is why it is so wonderful to have people like George who are led to want to be tested to be able to donate to strangers if needed. That is a real step in faith to do this for others. I so admire him for being a true servant of God in this way.

Our stories are quite different; everyone's story is, but knowing God is in control and has led many thousands of people to take this step for either a relative or a stranger is a true testament to the wonderful power of our God. He can open our eyes to things that we can do for others in diverse ways. Let us be ever mindful of the needs of others and take that step of faith and offer to be of help in some way.

"And do not forget to do good and share with others,
for with such sacrifices God is pleased."
– Hebrews 13:16 (ESV)

Bobbie:

The results of the two-day testing process arrived, and my son was approved to donate his kidney. Wow! I was amazed at the advancement of science over the years, and I still couldn't believe my son wanted to give up one of his organs for someone he had never met. The same thoughts flooded my mind like when he first expressed his interest in the living organ donation process. *What if he needed a kidney donation later in life? How will this affect his health and ability to care for his family? What if this limits the physical activity he is used to doing?* Again, in some way I had hoped this would go away. I hoped this was a fad that would fade with time and chalk it up to another idea of my son's that wouldn't endure the test of time.

Nonetheless, he remained committed to the cause and expressed his desire to continue to go forth, reassuring me that he had the ability to call off the process at any time. He could even call off the process the day of surgery if for some reason he wasn't confident in the process. The MUSC makes it clear that living donors have the authority to direct their surgery plans. The ball is in their court, and I suppose that brought me a little bit of comfort. I continued to hope that even though he had gone through the process to this point, he would stop it before it came time for surgery. The good news coming from the test was that his kidneys were healthy, and there wasn't anything found of concern. My son was declared healthy and able to become a living kidney donor.

I continued to research the process myself and was comforted on the improvements of the living donation surgeries over the years.

Recovery time had been shortened from months to weeks because of smaller incisions. In fact, at MUSC in Charleston, they now perform operations with robots controlled by surgeons for even more precise movements. I learned how most living organ donors continue to live a healthy and productive life well after their donation surgery. I read about living organ donors returning to running marathons, climbing mountains, and swimming in oceans. They lived their lives much like how they had before surgery, and they continued to do so decades after their donation surgery. This knowledge brought me comfort but still didn't change the fact that this was my son considering the donation process. This process moved too close to home for my comfort.

The waiting would continue even though he was approved to donate because he had chosen to commit his kidney to a specific person. He became aware of the need in this person's life because of his job. He works as a news photographer at a local tv station and people are always sending story ideas to the newsroom.

His awareness came when a family member wanted to make people aware of the kidney donation needed by their sister. He was so moved he decided to ask his kidney go to this particular person. The donation process is complicated, and many factors must line up for a donation to continue. He didn't directly match with who he felt led to commit his organ donation, so this delayed the process. Nurses told him since he wasn't a direct match, they would try to match him with someone else who also had someone who could donate to his original recipient. This delay also brought me comfort because I thought, *Maybe he will still forget about this idea and walk away from it.*

George:

On March 11, 2021, I received a call from MUSC saying I was approved to be a living kidney donor. This news came about one week after completing the testing and meeting with doctors about the potential of becoming a living kidney donor. I received the test results of my various kidney scans on the second day of my visit to MUSC on March 5, 2021, and everything looked good. Doctors, nurses, and support staff don't make their decision to approve a living donor on the test results alone. A lot of discussion about family medical history, mental health, and donor support system takes place as well.

All the pieces need to be in place before a potential living donor becomes an approved living donor. This is why discussion with your family, friends, co-workers, and work supervisors are important. Ultimately, the decision to donate is yours, but you are going to need help through the recovery process, and you will need to take time off from work. MUSC educated me on the support options available during recovery at the time and encouraged me to take as much time off work as I could. My surgery would most likely be on a Wednesday, and I remember initially thinking how I would be able to be back to work in a limited capacity the following Monday. Thankfully, I was quickly educated on the reality of the need to take at least two weeks off, but they recommended four to six weeks. I took four weeks off from work, and I am grateful I was able to do so. Before testing began, I was connected with the National Living Donor Assistance Center (NLDAC) that has been helping potential living donors and those who have completed a donation for over fifteen years. The NLDAC will help pay for travel, hotel, and food for you and a companion throughout the testing and surgery process. They may also be able to help offset loss of wages because of time away from work during surgery recovery. As a potential living donor and throughout the entire process, help is available to you, but most importantly, you need to identify who will be caring for you after surgery should you choose to become a living donor.

For me this was a humbling experience because I realized I had to ask for help. I don't like asking for help. I don't know many people who do. I believe it is in our nature to want to *appear strong* as if we *have it all together*, when in reality, we may be screaming inside saying, *I don't know what to do!* I had to have open discussions with my employer about being away for a month. I had to be open to the concerns and thoughts of my family and friends, and I also had to ask for their support through surgery recovery. I wasn't sure myself if I should go through with becoming a living kidney donor, but I did know I wanted to help and serving a greater purpose always remained before me. I have already said our blessings in life are not meant to be limited to our own use. They are meant to be shared with family, friends, and ultimately the world. I believe we are meant to be used as vessels of God's goodness, mercy, compassion, and love. We are blessed to bless others; we acquire to distribute, and we give not expecting to receive in return. This doesn't mean we give everything away, but it does mean we make everything available. Before becoming a living donor, I had to consider my responsibilities to my family and workplace. What kind of impact would surgery have on my role as financial provider to my family? How would my month long absence affect my workplace? Who would help me get out of bed if I couldn't get out myself after surgery? The transplant team at MUSC pushed me to ask these questions and seek the answers.

This time of discovery included another release of my will into God's hands. I had to remain humble. I had to listen, and I had to consider what I was hearing. In a way this pumped the brakes on my hopes and anticipation of wanting to help. I wanted to help now, but I was having to wait. I listened with great consideration to those who encouraged me to donate and those who didn't and gave their views. I had loving conversations with family who wanted me to be sure I evaluated all sides of becoming a living donor. I remembered they were seeking my best interest, not only for me, but for my children as well. The process of kidney transplant surgery has come a long way in the past one hundred years, but a surgery is still a surgery, and we should avoid the use of the word routine for any of them. My decision to move forward with the donation process after being approved to donate came from my faith in the faithfulness of God, the support of my family, friends, and employer, and my desire to help. My eyes were opened to the need, and it had been made clear I was able to help. Now the question was, *Who will I help?*

I wrestled with this question, *Who will I help?* Throughout the donation testing process, I had seen a need for living kidney donation. I asked myself if any of these people were specifically for me or should I become a *good Samaritan donor?* I was conflicted and unsure, so I asked God through prayer. I asked others to pray as well and ultimately decided to move forward in faith for one specific person. I had never met this person but knew she was a mother and wanted to continue to live so she could raise her family and have the freedom a healthy body can give. I was not a direct match for this woman, but because I said I would, for her this opened up more opportunities for her to receive a kidney through a kidney paired donation or kidney exchange. Basically, doctors would look to match me with someone else who would have a match available to whom I was hoping to donate. I was connected with this family and was able to talk with her brother about the news of being approved to donate and how I believed I was to be connected to his sister. We were both very excited and had great hopes for what was to come. We praised God for His faithfulness and love toward us, and we prayed for the days, weeks, and what became months ahead as we waited for a match.

I am not able to fully comprehend the waiting process for someone in need of a kidney, but I believe I shared a sliver of it while waiting to donate. From the moment of deciding to donate to a specific person and having to wait for a kidney-paired donation, I looked at every phone call ring with anticipation, especially calls from numbers I didn't recognize, and wondered if the call would be about setting a surgery date. I continued to live my life and do what I normally did, but I did make plans more carefully with consideration to the possibility of a surgery being scheduled. As a potential donor, I had a lot of say on the scheduling of testing and possible surgery, but I knew I didn't want someone in need to have to wait any longer than he/she already had waited. While waiting for testing, I witnessed the joy of those who were once on dialysis and facing death who received a kidney and had the hope of life restored within them. There was laughter in the waiting area as stories were swapped about life before transplant and life after and the profound impact receiving a kidney made. I wanted to help bring that change into someone's life as soon as possible.

Again, I had to release my desires to God and my timing unto His. I choose to do this because when I trust in God's timing, the outcome will be far better than I can imagine. God will be glorified, and my faith and others will be encouraged. A great illustration of this truth comes from John 11. John 11 tells us about the relationship Jesus had with Martha, her sister Mary, and their brother Lazarus. Martha and Mary knew Jesus; they were following Him through His ministry and listening to His teachings. When their brother Lazarus became ill, they went to Jesus to ask for help. In John 3:11 (NKJV) they say, "Lord, behold, he whom You love is sick." Something strange happens after this. What do you and I do under most circumstances when we hear someone we love is sick? We immediately go and see how we can help. Jesus remained where He was for a few more days. This doesn't make sense, does it? In fact, John 11:17 (NKJV) says, "So when Jesus came, He found that (Lazarus) had already been in the tomb four days." Jesus delayed long enough that sick Lazarus was now dead and buried. Certainly, Martha and Mary would have every right to be upset and disappointed with Jesus, but they didn't allow the circumstance to take away their communion with Christ. Martha boldly goes to Jesus before He arrives in town in John 11:21-22 (NKJV) saying, "Lord, if You had been here, my brother would not have died. But even now I know that whatever You ask of God, God will give You." Jesus replies in John 11:23 (NKJV) saying, "Your brother will rise again." Through the death of Lazarus, Jesus reveals Himself as the resurrection and the life. Jesus says in John 11:25-26 (NKJV), "I am the resurrection and the life. He who believes in Me, though he may die, he shall live. And whoever lives and believes in Me shall never die." This truth would not be revealed if Lazarus hadn't died. Martha, Mary, those around them, and Lazarus himself wouldn't see Jesus as an overcomer of death; they would have only seen Him as a healer of sickness. Through the power of God, Martha and Mary see Lazarus walk out of the tomb.

They see even the power of death doesn't have domain over the power of God. God chose to reveal this through the death of Lazarus so we may also know we can trust Him. Even when it appears like there is a delay in our prayers, hopes, and requests, we can have peace knowing with God all things are possible. Even someone dead and buried for four days can be called back to life. Why? Because maybe God wants to reveal Himself in a new way to you and me. Jesus knew He was heard by God but says in John 11:42 (NKJV), "And I know that You always hear Me, but because of the people who are standing by I said this, that they may believe that You sent Me." God does the impossible so there can be no doubt of credit being returned to Him. John 11:43 (NKJV) says, "Now when (Jesus) had said these things, He cried with a loud voice, 'Lazarus, come forth!'" He who had died came out. He who was once sick, dead, and buried now walked. You wouldn't believe it unless you saw it, and many did and shared their story, and we have the benefit of reading it today.

We learn about the compassion God has for us through John 11:1-44 (NKJV). Jesus weeps as He stands in front of the closed tomb of Lazarus. God knows all about our feelings of loss and our struggle to understand why sickness comes and why it may last until death. He has compassion for you and me and everyone else and wants us to trust Him. Trust in His timing; trust in His plans because they lead to life. This is what I did because I could read about how delays led to blessings bigger than what anyone could imagine. The delays led to blessings that not only impacted those immediately affected but also the world.

Choose to not worry while waiting and look to God. Know God hears you and loves you. You, too, may say to Him in a time of sickness, "Lord, behold, the one whom You love is sick." You too may say to Him in a time of trial, "Lord, behold, the one whom You love doesn't understand and is losing hope. Father, we have lots of questions in this life and look to You for answers. Thank you for the answers you have already given through the examples of Scripture. Thank you for Your choice to love us beyond what we can see and help us to not worry but wait well. Help us to resist the desire to take all matters into our own hands and utilize our own plans. May we continually turn them over to You so they may be used for Your glory."

Jesus called upon Martha to roll the stone away from Lazarus's tomb in John 11:39 (NJKV), and although she initially protested, with help she did. We want to be those who obey because obedience leads to blessing. May we help each other to obey and may we remain still until called upon to obey. In Jesus' name Amen.

A Prayer for the Findings:

What do you do when you receive unexpected results? What do you do when the answer you receive is not the answer you desire? Do you react out of your disappointment or remain steadfast in your convictions? You do have a choice in your response to unexpected results. Remember our God can do anything, and He has already done everything for You to know Him through Jesus Christ. Cry out to God in faith because He does hear you, and He will respond. Trust in His response and remain present in His presence.

Jesus gives an unfavorable response to a woman in Mark 7:24-30. The woman is identified as a Greek, a Syro-Phoenician by birth in verse 26. She was not Jewish, and at that specific time in history, had no claim to the promises of God. She kept asking Jesus to heal her daughter. She came to Him and fell at His feet! But how does Jesus respond? He says, (NKJV) "Let the children be filled first, for it is not good to take the children's bread and throw it to the little dogs."

The language Jesus uses here may seem harsh, but He is making a point and in other words says, "I am not here for you now; my dealings are with the nation of Israel." How does the woman respond? She doesn't get angry, she doesn't walk away in disgust, and she doesn't curse God. She remains present in the conversation and boldly says this in verse 28, "Yes, Lord, yet even the little dogs under the table eat from the children's crumbs." She agrees with Jesus but adds that even the dogs get a little something from the table. They don't starve and feed on the crumbs. Jesus responds in verse 29, "For this saying go your way; the demon has gone out of your daughter."

Even if you aren't receiving the reports or results you had hoped for, remain present with God. Remain honest and bold before His throne of grace and mercy. This woman remained bold. She didn't walk away. She continued the conversation and operated out of her conviction that even though she wasn't from the nation of Israel, she was a benefactor of their blessings. You are a benefactor of the blessings of God through Jesus Christ. His will is for you to press on through negative responses and trust in Him to make the wrongs right. Don't walk away from God but remain present in His presence. Ask questions and be bold in your prayers.

Father God, may I always see You for Who You are. You are good, You are kind, You are powerful, and You are God. I am under Your covering, under the shadow of Your wings, and You will take care of me. May my conviction of Your goodness come from Your Word and not from unexpected negative results in my life. I recognize the negative results are temporary, and Your goodness is eternal. Lead me through this trial and may I be bold in my interactions with You. May I speak from faith in Your goodness and trust in Your deliverance. I declare I am a child of God through Jesus Christ, and I will remain present with my Father through this trial in Jesus' name, Amen!

"There is an appointed time for everything,
A time for every event under heaven."
– **Ecclesiastes 3:1 (NASB)**

Part 6 - The Surgery

Yvette:

After all the worrying, waiting, testing, and finally the results, the day came when the transplant was needed. The surgery date was set. The previous day we were to be at the hospital for a final test, a bleeding test to ensure the platelets were functioning correctly and to determine how quickly the blood clotted from the time the patient was cut to the time the bleeding completely stopped. During that test Jake experienced a vagal response, which involved the central nervous system, the peripheral nervous system, and the cardiovascular system being compromised. This caused an abrupt drop in blood pressure and a sudden reduction in the heart rate. This does not happen to everyone, but it was Jake's body reacting to what was being done to him—being cut to watch the blood flow and clot.

The blood vessels in his legs widened, which caused blood to pool in his legs, causing him to pass out and his heart to stop beating for a brief time.

Due to this happening, they chose to admit him right then and keep an eye on him the rest of the day and overnight to make sure nothing would keep the surgery from happening the next morning. Being his mother, I chose to stay with him all night to make sure he

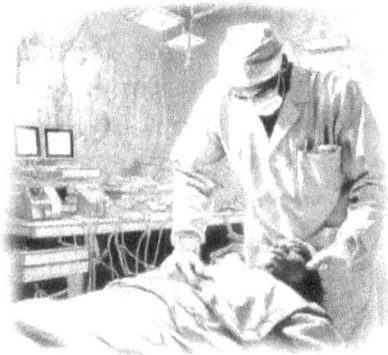

was okay, and that way, I would already be there in the morning to be prepped and ready for the transplant to begin.

Our family and friends arrived bright and early the next morning. It was September 13, 1994. During this time, being a donor was a different experience than it is today. Today it is a less invasive operation and less recovery time for the donor, which is wonderful for those who wish to be an organ donor.

After saying our "see you later" goodbyes to our family, Jake and I were taken to our opposite operating rooms, and we had a moment of connection with each other, expressing no fear but peace and calm about what would take place. I prayed my family waiting had the same peace and calm too. I knew Gary was praying for both of us. His thoughts would be, *Please don't let my son die, and please protect my wife.* I knew Jason would be worried about us both, and Lori shared when asked what her thoughts were on surgery day that her thoughts were *all over the place* from positive to negative. She said she thought about her daddy and how he was doing. He is the strength of the family, but on that day, she was concerned that maybe he was more worried than he wanted everyone to believe. She knew that with his head hung and eyes closed that he was talking to God, asking for all to be well, and there was a sense of comfort to her too, knowing he was talking to God. She was worried about Jason too and if he was truly okay or if he needed her. She felt he was just numb, and she began to pray too. She shared later that as she prayed, she had a sense of calmness knowing all would be fine. And she needed to be strong for her family. Jake had been very brave through it all, and for the most part, was very positive about the outcome, although she knew he was worried about me more than himself. All in all, she had hope, and felt some relief that Jake was finally going to feel better after being so sick.

The prayers of all who were praying for us were felt, and we had a blessed assurance that all would be well; we knew we were being held in the palm of God's hand and that He would be directing the surgeons' hands through every second of both surgeries. We would both be fine throughout the surgeries; we were well taken care of by the doctors and nurses that day.

The surgeries would begin with one of the surgeons placing

me on my right side with my head and feet slightly lower than the rest of my body to make the removal of the kidney easier for them. The left kidney is preferred to be removed for the transplant because of the implantation advantages of having longer vessels and being more accessible to remove.

Remember, this is 1994, so the surgery was more invasive then. It is done laparoscopic now so not as much cutting is involved as then. I remind you of this so you will be assured that it is so much easier to be a donor in this day and age, so do not let it keep you from considering to become a donor. I just felt I should share my experience then to compare the *then and now*.

The surgeon made an approximately twelve-inch incision, starting on the front of my belly and going up to my ribs. After removing the necessary muscle, fat, and tissue out of the way, the twelfth rib was cut to provide more room for the process of taking the kidney out.

(Ironically, after hearing this, I thought about how God removed a rib from Adam to create Eve—with God, all things are possible.)

Next, the tube that carries the urine from the kidney to the bladder and blood vessels was cut away from the kidney as the kidney was removed and then taken to be prepared for Jake to receive the new kidney. The procedure to remove my kidney took about three hours to perform.

Jake had been prepared by his surgeon, making incisions in the lower part of his abdomen on his right side, where the new kidney would be placed. They did not remove the old kidneys, as was the practice, unless there had been any infection, kidney stones, or anything that would have caused a problem during the operation. Because of his disease, his kidneys were shriveled up like raisins, so it was no problem leaving them.

The new kidney was placed in him just above his leg after the blood vessels that had been removed with it were attached to the blood vessels in his abdomen. Then the ureter tube of the kidney would be attached to his bladder. Although this procedure sounds so simple compared to removing it, the surgery was done with less room to move things around with smaller instruments and took around three hours to complete. Of course, to Jake and me, it seemed like no time at all had passed when it was over and we awoke, but our family and friends went through many long hours praying and waiting to hear the results.

After recovery and being moved to our rooms, we both were feeling great. I had expected to be in a room right next door to Jake but was surprised to learn that I was at the other end of the hall. After asking about that, I was told that it was for our own good. The key to getting better is getting up and moving around. If we were next door, it would not take much effort to walk there, but this way we would have much more walking to do to see each other. That was smart of them. It didn't take long before I just had to see how Jake was doing with my own eyes. So, I got up to make my way down to check on him.

I took my pillow and held it against my side to make it more comfortable and hobbled right down to his room! He looked so wonderful. His color was back to a healthy glow; he was smiling and sharing with me how everything seemed so much better already. My heart was filled with thanksgiving when after I said it is so great what they can do with God's direction and that I felt this kidney would serve him well for a long time, he replied, "Oh, I know it will, Mom. When I was in the bathroom just now, I gave a little prayer of thanks, and I heard the angels singing that all was well. I have many years of good health ahead for me."

"But let all who take refuge in you be glad, let them ever sing for joy. Spread your protection over them, that those who love your name may rejoice in you."
– Psalm 5:11 (NIV)

"Consider it pure joy, my brothers, and sisters, whenever you face trials of many kinds because you know that the testing of your faith produces perseverance. Let perseverance finish its work so that you may be mature and complete, not lacking anything. If any of

you lacks wisdom, you should ask God,
who gives generously to all without
finding fault, and it will be given to you.
But when you ask, you must believe and not doubt,
because the one that doubts is like a wave
of the sea, blown and tossed by the wind.
That person should not expect to receive anything
from the Lord. Such a person is double-minded
and unstable in all they do."
– James 1:2-8 (NIV)

The key to making it through tough times is having faith in God. We must ask in faith and not doubt God's goodness. He truly wants to give us what we need, and we must pray and ask for wisdom and expect God to deliver it. If we don't, we are being controlled by our circumstances. We are being double-minded. One moment we trust God, and the next moment we doubt. When we have faith always during our trials, we can ask God and He will hear us.

Bobbie:
The day of surgery has come. I can't believe it, but I am not surprised. My son has always had a sweet caring side to him, but these past few years he has become more caring and compassionate toward the needs of others. I believe his compassion and kindness has brought him to this point. I have come with him as a loving and supportive mother. I have committed to being his caregiver during this process, as well as my husband who made the trip from Myrtle Beach to Charleston too. Nonetheless, I do not like seeing my son go through this process. I am scared and don't want to see his gift of a kidney affect his long-term health and life experience. *He has responsibilities and two daughters to continue to raise. What if something happens and he can't return to work or a normal way of life? Will I have to take care of him and my granddaughters?* These thoughts ran through my mind, but as I said I was committed to being here for my son. This is a beautiful, compassionate, loving act

of kindness he was doing, but to me there must be another way to show his desire to love others. *Does his version of loving others have to be this way?* I had hoped he would call off this process well before this day, but here we were in Charleston, walking to MUSC at 5 AM so he could become a living kidney donor.

Peace and quiet filled the main lobby of the hospital at 5 AM. There weren't many people around as we walked in and checked in. We waited in the lobby, and I mentioned to my son he could still turn around. He said he felt well and wanted to proceed. His name was called, and a band was placed around his right wrist. The surgery became more real as every minute passed. I was freaking out inside but tried to keep my appearance together. A few tears fell down my face as we left the lobby and proceeded toward the next steps in the process. I was not sure why I felt this way except for maybe fear of the unknown. I was amazed by the advancements in medical science over the past fifty years, especially in the area of organ donation, but I still had doubts. Surgery was still surgery. Doctors were still opening up a human being, moving around, and removing parts that didn't need to be moved around or removed in my opinion. I suppose if this was for someone I knew or a family member, I wouldn't have been as shaken by this process. I just didn't want my son to die or have a hindered life from health problems because of this gift. I thought, *He doesn't need to do this, and no one is asking him to, but he has decided to step forward to have a kidney removed. I really don't know where he comes up with these ideas sometimes, but he is my son, and I love him, and I am here to support him.*

I got to be with him after he had changed into the hospital gown and nurses and techs had finished preparing him for surgery. I was nervous, and he confessed some nerves, as well, but his spirits were high, which encouraged me. I recorded a video of him lying in bed with a smile on his face as he gave a thumbs up and said, "Ready to go!" I was proud, worried, and fearful all at the same time. I was proud of my son for stepping up and helping someone in need. He knew this truth and was also appreciative of the sacrifice my husband and I had made to be here with him that day. I don't think he could believe he was here either. This day had been long anticipated and had now arrived. There had been so many moving parts, and not one of them had gone off the rails to cause a delay in the process. He was here in the hospital, prepped for kidney donation surgery, and about to be wheeled into the operating room. This was really happening. Oh my gosh! The time had come and the nurse wheeled him away. I made my way to the waiting area. I looked forward to the next few hours passing quickly, and the next time I would see my son, he would be one kidney lighter.

The waiting area was quiet and cold like most hospitals. I had come prepared with a bag full of support materials including a blanket and book. The surgery update system includes a color code system to keep families updated on the progress of their loved ones. My son was given a number at check in, and this number showed up on the screen with a color assignment. Each color corresponded to a specific stage of the surgery process. For the most part, all the colors were good, but there was a *gray* that disturbed me. I prayed the gray stayed away because it meant deceased or something similar. As long as I didn't see gray next to my son's number, I was happy! I shared this with him later, and we still talk about it today. I hope no one ever has to see gray by a loved one's number, and I wonder why they even have it on the screen.

Anyway, I was thankful for the continued updates on the progress of my son's surgery, and I believe the staff made it as efficient as possible. Eventually, I saw his status moved to recovery, and at one point, his surgeon even came out to speak with me personally. I appreciated her desire to communicate personally, and she shared great words of comfort and confidence that all had gone as planned with my son's surgery. Wow! The surgery was done and my son now had one kidney. I couldn't believe it and called my husband and shared the news with friends and family. What began with an idea from a sticker on the back of a car had now come to my son lying in a recovery room from donating a kidney.

Not long after speaking with the doctor, I was able to see my son in his room. This is where we stayed until he checked out of the hospital, which would hopefully have been the next day. Of course, he was tired, and we didn't talk much at first, but it was good to see him on the other side of surgery!

I am still amazed at the entire process and thankful I could be there with him on that day. There are so many variables to this process, and I was overjoyed seeing my son come through the other side. Like a checklist, I checked off the parts that had been passed. The recovery began, and I hoped I never had to be in a hospital room with my son again.

George:

The waiting, praying, and preparation culminated on September 7, 2022. The MUSC staff scheduled me to arrive at the hospital at 5 AM. I didn't sleep much the night before because of prescribed surgery preparations, but that didn't stop me from being excited.

My mother and I walked to the hospital since we stayed a few blocks away. We talked about the surgery and took a picture in front of the main entrance. While we waited to check in, I looked around and wondered if my recipient was in the waiting area with me. I didn't know to whom I was donating, but I did know he or she were having surgery in the same hospital. I wondered how I would respond to the anesthesia since I heard many different stories of how others responded in the past. Only time would tell, but I was confident in the entire process because of the years of study and dedication to the process others had put forth throughout the decades of transplant surgery. I knew for sure whatever happened would be covered by the grace of God, and I had peace.

I also had to answer one question over and over again, "Why are you here today?" At one point, I joked with one of the nurses and said, "I am here to have my teeth cleaned." They laughed and then asked again so they could hear me say, "I am here to donate my kidney." What an amazing advancement in the understanding of the human body that we are able to *swap parts* from one person to another. James 1:17 (NKJV) says, "Every good gift and every perfect gift is from above, and comes down from the Father of lights, with whom there is no variation or shadow of turning." God gives life and brings order out of chaos.

In God's time, He brought forth His son Jesus to save us all who were far from Him, and in His time, He revealed a way for man to help another through the blessing of organ transplant surgery. I had great hope that morning and great hope today because our God creates with the end in mind. This world came to be through His Word and His creativity, and attention to detail is witnessed through nature and our lives. The time had come for my kidney to be gifted to another in need, and I was thankful to be able to be a part of such significant life change.

I believe thanksgiving to God really carried me through that morning. I was thankful to make it to surgery day without complications, thankful to have my family with me, and specifically my mother with me in the waiting room, and thankful to be healthy enough to donate. I try not to take anything for granted and especially health. Move and exercise as much as you can while you can because a healthy body stands a much better chance against any attack than an unhealthy one. Use what you are able to use with hope that more ability will come as you persist in health. I don't know why some can eat bread all day and not gain a pound and some eat one slice of bread and scream, but I do know we are all here for a purpose, and we are here to help one another. I believe part of my purpose was to share my health and kidney. Through faith in Jesus and His promise to never leave or forsake me, I walked into the hospital with my head held high. This was going to be a great day of new experiences and celebrations!

You are here for a purpose, and God's plans for our lives are always bigger than we can envision and accomplish on our own. Again, I love Ephesians 3:20-21 (NKJV) that says, "Now to Him who is able to do exceedingly abundantly above all that we ask or think, according to the power that works in us, to Him be glory in the church by Christ Jesus to all generations, forever and ever. Amen."

This encourages me, and I hope it encourages you as well. I don't see the entire picture, but I know the Painter and the Painter is AWESOME! I needed help from many people to get me to this day. I needed encouragement and support from my family. I needed to have the support of work for the time off. I needed help in the care of my daughters while I was away and during recovery. I needed and help was available, praise the Lord! The staff at MUSC were great guides in finding help where I couldn't find it myself. These are additional reasons why I had such great confidence the day of surgery.

I have vivid memories waiting to be wheeled back into surgery and vivid memories of waking up, but I don't remember anything about the surgery itself other than being wheeled into the OR (operating room). They moved me from the bed to the operating table and that was it. Next thing I knew I was waking up in the recovery area. I have discovered I do well with anesthesia, and I remember being quite happy waking up. I prayed with my nurse who then quickly announced I was ready to go to my room. So, there I was in the early afternoon in my room on the road to recovery from kidney surgery. Amazing!

Before surgery, nurses shared with me various reactions donor patients have to surgery. Some will stay an extra night or two after surgery to rest and have help managing pain. Others will be out of bed the next day with clothes changed and ready to go home. I wanted to be the out of bed patient. I wanted to be up and walking around, ready to meet my recipient (and I hoped they wanted to meet me too) and out the door by the afternoon. The encouragement the nurses and doctors gave me really helped prepare me for what may come. Although as I continued to wake up in my hospital room, I wasn't seeing how anyone could be up and walking around the next day. I was tired and in pain. I also had a catheter connected to my bladder, so I didn't have to get up to use the bathroom. That was the most bizarre situation and one I wasn't expecting, but I understand why it was done. I had no interest in getting up from my bed in those immediate hours after surgery anyways. I slept a lot and ate a little. My loving family came to visit me and sit with me, and I know they were thankful my recovery had begun.

While I slept, I continued to envision the next day and being up and walking around to meet my recipient. Everyone involved in surgery wanted to meet each other, and the plan was to welcome each other in the late morning on Thursday, September 8th. I rested and looked forward to our meeting.

The staff at MUSC deeply cares about each patient and each

patient has a nurse and nurse aide assigned to him/her on a rotating schedule. I had peace knowing I was held in the loving arms of my Father in heaven, and it was evident through the nursing staff. I never felt alone in my room after surgery, and this strengthened my desire to get up and get moving. I wanted to get up; I wanted to move; I wanted to shower and change clothes; I wanted to meet whoever received my donated kidney. By God's grace my pain decreased, and my strength returned. I began sitting up and taking steps toward the bathroom. Little by little I made forward progress early the next day (like 5 AM early) and was beginning to feel like I could be the one who could be up, in changed clothes, and walking around free from a catheter and IV.

A few hours past 5 AM, my catheter was removed, and I attempted to take a shower and shave. Every step I had taken before then gave me confidence to keep going. The water flowed over my aching body and helped to further increase my strength. I was going to be the one to walk around after surgery! Praise God because I didn't see this happening hours before. My next feat was drinking a cup of coffee, and after that point, I was like, "Let's go!" My favorite moments in my hospital room were seeing my family with me and getting to meet the nursing staff. I am an encourager and loved hearing the pursuits of the nurses' aides especially. Most of them were in nursing school and had plans to become qualified nurses upon graduation from their courses. They, too, are encouragers and help to bring healing to those in need. I am so grateful for the love and care of the MUSC nursing staff. If you pursue this calling to become a living organ donor, you will find yourself in similar loving hands.

I brought my Bible and spent time with the Lord in the early hours, giving Him praise and thanks for leading me through every step of my donation journey. I knew the best was yet to come with being able to meet my recipient and everyone else involved in the kidney donor chain surgeries. My family had grown exponentially by the grace of God. I often write a sentence or two in a journal on a daily basis as I read God's word and reflect on the meaning and application to my daily life. I looked back in my journal from September 7th and 8th, 2022, and didn't find too much other than

"Blessed is the man who trusts in the LORD" from Psalm 2 on September 7th and a note to read Psalm 8 from September 8th.

Psalm 8 begins and ends with, "O LORD, our Lord. How excellent is Your name in all the earth" (NKJV)! This is a short Psalm compared to others with only nine verses, but those nine verses are power packed with revelation of God's character. Nine times the Psalm talks about the work of God. Verses begin with "You have" seven times in reference to the work God has done through His loving process of creation. Psalm 8 gives glory to God and recognizes Him as the source of life. Because of God, we are here today, and because of God, medical advancements have occurred to the level they are today. Every positive, life giving, and rewarding human achievement that has been obtained to this day is a gift of God. Psalm 8 culminates in verses 4 and 5, "What is man that You are mindful of him, And the son of man that You visit him? For You have made him a little lower than the angels. And You have crowned him with glory and honor." God crowned humanity with glory and honor not because of what we do for Him. He crowns us because He loves us. There is nothing we need to do or can do to achieve this crowning. The only thing you can do is receive it with joy and trust God to have done it because He has said it. I also wrote this in my journal on September 8th: "I'm getting stronger every day by the power of the Spirit. The Lord is my strength and salvation. I will stand on the rock knowing I can't be shaken. Because of what is spoken, I believe."

"He comforts us in all our affliction, so that we may
be able to comfort those who are in any affliction."
– 2 Corinthians 1:4a (ESV)

A Second Transplant Needed

Yvette:

After seventeen good years of the kidney working that I donated to my son Jake, it looked like the disease had been slowly working on destroying the new kidney. He was beginning to feel bad and becoming sick easier than before. He began seeing a nephrologist to keep watch on how the kidney was functioning and checking the creatinine levels, which would give indication when it would be time for another transplant. Jacob's twin brother, Jason, was tested and found to be a great match for this second transplant. We wanted to have everything in order and ready when it was time so the surgery could be done right away and, hopefully, keep Jake from having to be on dialysis and continuing to get increasingly sick. Jake shared how God had blessed him with another living, related donor who was his twin brother whom he loved and had a strong bond with, but he was a little worried that he would be putting another family member in danger.

Jason had no problem saying yes to being the donor for the second transplant that his brother would need. As he had stated when asked about it, "It was an easy yes. I didn't see any reason not to do it; he needed it! It felt like a natural response to help someone you love who is in need." He had been concerned thinking about his two children and contemplating what might happen if they ever had the same need, but he quickly decided that he could not live under a *what if* type scenario. His brother needed help now. When asked what gave him confidence in proceeding with the donation process, his reply was, "First is the sound belief that everything would be ok. We've had the grace of God present in our lives since I can remember, so I guess my thought was that no matter what happened we were all going to be taken care of. And then that extended out to the rest of my family. We all would be there for each other to make sure that the love and care that exists between us all is never absent."

We had hoped that this next experience with the transplant would go as smoothly as the first one did, but as it turned out, Jake had many hard years before the transplant was finally scheduled.

Several unforeseen health problems occurred as his kidney failure progressed. It seemed that his immune system was not able to fight off any type of sickness at all, and each time he went for a check-up, there seemed to be another potential problem delaying the surgery. He had to be hospitalized a couple of times due to health problems and was eventually put on dialysis.

It was very heartbreaking to see Jake go through such a struggle, especially when there was a healthy living donor there and ready. If his immune system had not been so weak, the transplant could have happened right away. There should never be a delay if there is a living donor.

I am not putting blame on anyone because of this long delay, but as a mother, there are times when our gut just tells us that something isn't right.

Jake said that the dialysis was making it hard to feel normal. He was tired all the time and felt drained and also felt like the end of his life was coming much sooner than he had wanted, which was to see his son grow up; they were enjoying spending lots of time together, and he wanted more time with him to see him grow up.

After Jake shared with us that he was losing hope and didn't think he was going to make it to be able to have another transplant and asked us to please take care of his son, I could not rest without doing something.

My husband Gary and I were getting very concerned about what was going on and began to doubt the care Jake was getting from the local nephrologist. It didn't seem right that Jake was being passed around from one doctor to another and not getting well enough for the transplant.

Jake's comment when I voiced this concern was that he wasn't the only patient the doctor had, and he was very busy with them all. I tried to continue to be patient, but this was my son, and I felt I was supposed to do something now! Whatever I could do to make things better for him was what I wanted to do.

Thankfully, God led me to make a call to one of the doctors that had been on the team when I was his donor in 1994. After explaining the situation to the nurse, we were granted an appointment quickly and went to see him. Upon entering his office and seeing my face, he asked what was wrong. My reply was, "I think they are going to let my son die."

Jake and I explained everything that had been going on. The fact was he had a living donor, his twin brother. The fact was he was just getting increasingly sick. The fact was he was on dialysis. And then the fact was Jake shared that he didn't think he would make it to even be able to get a transplant in time to save him.

By the grace of God, this doctor took Jake as his patient without delay, and within two months, the surgeries were scheduled. I do not know the reason for such a long delay. I did not mention the doctor whom I had lost hope in and do not know if they investigated. I do not know if Jake had been by some accident put on a waiting list for a donor, like I have discovered can happen. None of that was my concern now. My concern was giving thanks to our God Who had made sure that Jake was now going to be taken care of even though it was a tough road to travel.

I share all of this not to scare anyone, but to remind us that life happens. We won't always understand when there are problems and heartaches, but we must never forget that God is with us even when we don't realize it. When we are waiting for answers, and it seems almost too late, God understands our feelings and deeply cares for our pain. He bears our burdens when we are weak.

> *"The Lord is close to the brokenhearted*
> *and saves those who are crushed in spirit."*
> **– Psalm 34:18 (NIV)**

So, Jake was finally at the hospital the night before the transplant, again being watched so nothing would go wrong that could delay this from happening. Gary and I and Jason and his wife Lisa were all staying in a hotel in Charlotte, so we could be there without any delays in the morning at 4:30 AM. We did not need to be there that early, but after waiting so long for this to finally happen, we were excited and happy to be there. We checked on Jake and spoke with the surgeons. We talked with Jason who said he was a little emotional but in a good way. He was thankful for the opportunity and confident of the outcome but a little scared because he was heading into something unknown, like I think we all might be if we are honest. Jake and Jason were prepped, and we were allowed to go in and have a last word and prayer before they were taken into the operating rooms. It was heartwarming to see both boys (well men--I will always call them my boys) smiling and showing no signs of being scared or worried. It took me back to the time I was lying there with Jake waiting all those years before, and I knew they both had that same peace knowing all would be well. God's presence was felt by all of us—Blessed Assurance!

As they were being wheeled away, with outstretched arms, they both told each other, "I love you Jake," "I love you too Jason." My heart still smiles when I think about that; there are no sweeter words for a parent to hear spoken between his/her thirty-six-year-old sons than that, knowing it was for that time and for always. Gary was emotional and shared that seeing the love they had for each other was overwhelming; he cried with joy. Lori said that when she heard that her brothers had told each other they loved each other before entering the surgery rooms, it sweetened the deal for her that everything would be okay with them. They were in there together, doing this together, and fighting for each other. It can't get much better than that!

The hours seemed like a lifetime before we knew they were doing well. Both surgeries had been a success, and the kidney began working at once and beautifully after Jake received it. The total time of both surgeries took about the same amount of time as before— three hours or so each, even with Jason's surgery being done by the laparoscopic method.

We were thrilled that the method had advanced to being done in this way, and Jason did not have such an invasive and more painful surgery to undergo. This surgery required an inch incision in the lower abdomen for the kidney to be removed and four smaller incisions to serve as ports for the instruments to enter along with a small scope (camera). I could not imagine how tedious it must have been for the surgeon to do this instead of having a wide-open space to move things around. The steadiness of a surgeon's hands during these operations leaves me in awe. I cannot even thread a needle to sew without trying over and over. God was surely in control.

Jake's surgery was performed in the same way it had been done before, via the traditional open surgery method. His recovery would be a little longer than the first time considering all that had happened up to the time of surgery and with him being older, but there would be no more dialysis and no more being sent to every kind of doctor every time he turned around. God is so good.

Seeing hope and wellness ahead instead of the pain and sorrow of before was so wonderful. Happy crying, even though it can make your face look ugly, took the place of our thankful words. We were rejoicing in the Lord. We could not express our thanks enough to the team of doctors and nurses and all involved in this glorious day.

> *"Rejoice always, pray continually, give*
> *thanks, in all circumstances; for this is*
> *God's will for you in Christ Jesus."*
> **– 1 Thessalonians 5:16-18 (NIV)**

Jason was released to go home first and Jake not too long after. Jason healed quickly and was back to his active life in no time: camping, biking, hiking, and fun with his family. Jake recovered soon and was very thankful that everything ended up well, and as he said, "I was glad to have another chance at life and hope I can continue to live and be a part of a loving family for many more years. God was with us, and we all pulled through."

When Jake was asked what he would like to share with those who are in a similar situation as he had been, he shared the following.

"I know that everyone deals with things in his/her own way. This is dependent on the situation they are in, how long they are waiting, and how close they are to God. All these factors set us up for a positive experience or one that can drain the life out of you. I know having strong ties to my religion, my family, my partner, and my friends helped me feel normal and that it was just something that was challenging me to be a better person. I think staying positive and having a good attitude is a strong ally to healing. You create certain chemicals in your body that produce emotions and reactions

in your chemical makeup. I do believe that those chemicals can help to strengthen your immune system and your body's reaction to those diseases. So, stay positive, pray, and keep your family close."

I am amazed at times at how smart my kids have become as they have grown. They teach me things all the time, and I am one blessed Mom. All three have more wisdom than I ever did at their age. God has been so good to our family.

Gary shared his thoughts when asked the same question that Jake was. "Whether you are a recipient or a donor, know that there is hope and healing ahead; have faith in your family's support, and love your doctors' healing abilities, and love your God! I am truly more convinced that God is and will always be there for His children."

As I write this book, it has been going on fourteen years now since Jake received the second kidney transplant. He is being given many more wonderful years to spend with his son Liam, who is now in college and sharing time with us all, his family who love him. I am praying and counting on this kidney to last him the rest of his very long life, God willing.

Out of curiosity, I did some reading about brothers giving brothers kidneys and found there are brothers living today who had the same experience in 1997. They were a perfect match also and both men are healthy and doing great to this day, which is going on forty-eight years ago.

I continued to research after reading that and found that the longest surviving kidney transplant patient from a sibling is fifty-six years. Who knows? Maybe my boys will be the new record holder for that, too, one day. It could very well happen if it is God's will. I pray however long He wills that both my boys stay healthy and happy always, and most importantly that they continue to love the Lord and grow in their faith and the Word of God.

"Trust in the Lord with all your heart, and do not lean on your own understanding. In all ways acknowledge Him, and He will make straight your paths."
– Proverbs 3:5-6 (ESV)

Jake – Final thoughts shared:

The first doctor I had contact with was a genuinely nice doctor who explained the process well to me and was very generous and transparent with me. I was able to be well prepared and recognize that the time for a transplant was getting closer after about two years of first finding out I would one day need one.

The doctor helped me not to worry; we would know when it was time to have it done before any harm was done to make it a more serious operation, and he explained that I could live a normal life with this diagnosis.

I was very blessed to have a living donor, my mother, who insisted on doing it for me, so the waiting process and wondering about it all was not hard like it must be for those who do not have a living donor. I was nervous for her and did not want her to give up any of her time with the rest of my family, but all went smoothly, and my family was there in every way through it all.

On the day of the surgery, we were not nervous and were treating it like just another day of getting where we needed to be to have done what needed to be done. It helped that by that time, I had accepted the process and just gave it all to God, like my mom had done everything throughout her life. The surgery was a success, and I was blessed to have a second chance, and I knew that and was thankful.

It changed me for the better. I took notice of things that I had not originally noticed. The beauty in the wind and the smell of cold versus hot days. I did not get angry easily, I cried more, and it felt good. I understood the fragility of life and am more affected by people's stories. I listen more carefully and take time to hear people and consider their feelings and situations. I know I have been given a special gift from God to have had not one, but two more chances at life.

Even though the second transplant had many challenges that the first one did not have, I cannot complain. My different experiences allow me to share with others and make them aware that life does have a variety of trials and tribulations that we will face. If all were rosy, we would not appreciate what God does for us, and we would be lost in this life. So, praise God, and love one another.

A Prayer for Surgeries:

You have heard the call of God over life. His voice brought you to life through Jesus Christ. You stepped forward in faith because You believe in our Father in Heaven Who created you and desires to meet all your needs. Jesus says He will never leave you or forsake you. Do not question this truth now, but instead keep Your focus on the presence of God and His goodness.

Consider the apostle Peter's reaction when he saw Jesus coming to the boat he was in during the middle of the night.

Matthew 14:26-28 (NKJV) says,

> *"And when the disciples saw Him walking on the sea,*
> *they were troubled, saying, 'It is a ghost!' And they cried*
> *out for fear. But immediately Jesus spoke to them, saying,*
> *'Be of good cheer! It is I; do not be afraid.' And Peter answered*
> *Him and said, 'Lord, if it is You, command me to come*
> *to You on the water.'"*

Jesus said "Come" to Peter, and Peter went. Peter stepped out of the boat in faith because he trusted and believed in Jesus as the son of God. Peter believed the power of Jesus' words and deeds. Peter walked on the water to go to Jesus!

Verses 30-33 show us what happened when Peter became distracted by the situation.

> *"But when he saw that the wind was boisterous,*
> *he was afraid; and beginning to sink he cried out, saying,*
> *'Lord, save me!' And immediately Jesus stretched out*
> *His hand and caught him, and he said to him,*
> *'O you of little faith, why did you doubt?' And when*
> *they got into the boat, the wind ceased. Then those*
> *who were in the boat came and worshipped Him,*
> *saying, 'Truly you are the Son of God.'"*

God is faithful to His calling, and we must remain focused on Him. Confess your emotions, your anxieties, and your fears, and they will not distract you from the call of God upon your life. Keep moving forward in faith, and do not doubt because Jesus will not let you fall. The waves may be big and the wind may be great but God is greater!

Father, I pray for the release of my emotions, anxieties, and fears into Your hands. Although I may feel troubled, I will go forward with confidence. I choose to focus on You and not the circumstances before me because You are greater. Thank You for bringing me to this moment in time, and may I rejoice for what is to come. I trust in You, and You will not let me fall! I have come to this day in faith and now my faith will lead me through as I focus on You. As I lie here before my surgery, may Your surpassing peace be upon me and those around me. You will not let me fall! In Jesus' name, Amen!

"The Lord sustains them on their sickbed
and restores them from their bed of illness."
– Psalm 41:3 (NKJV)

Part 7 - Post Operation

Yvette:

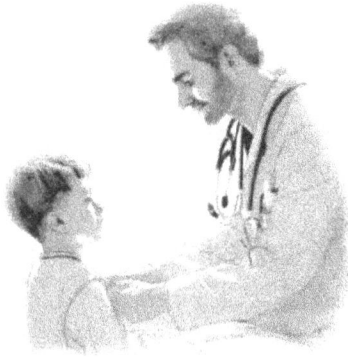

When the surgeries were over, all we wanted to do was to celebrate the doctors' good news that both surgeries were successful and all looked great. Thanking God was first for us and then family, and friends. We had so much to be thankful for and knew God was with us through each step of the way, guiding the surgeons' hands and helping the nurses do their job in the exact manner that needed to be done. This was all amazing.

Looking back, the whole process, from learning that our son needed a kidney transplant to the testing, to the many doctors' appointments to gauge and determine the exact time when he needed the transplant to take place (which in Jake's case was two years after hearing that news), to the wondering and worrying about everything known and unknown about it all, and to just trying to take it all in was monumental. We still had to continue with life all around us that needed to happen with the rest of the family. This made me realize that without God beside us each step of the journey, things would have been almost unbearable if we hadn't had the faith we had, along with all who were praying for us.

Having that faith and encouragement was needed even after

we were home. There were many adjustments after getting out of the hospital and returning home to continue the recovery without the nurses and doctors coming in to check on us. You realize that now you need to take care of certain things that were done for you before, and you need assurance and guidance from above.

> *"Do not neglect to do good and to share what you have,*
> *for such sacrifices are pleasing to God."*
> **– Hebrews 12:16 (ESV)**

Life After Transplants

Yvette and Family:

During the recovery period at home, you needed to be more aware of a different way of life that receiving an organ transplant will involve for the recipient. The body will need different treatment and more care in many ways. With Jake receiving a new kidney, the site where the kidney was placed was a spot that needed to be protected. It was now in his lower abdomen just above his leg. He needed to be aware of being gentler and not doing any rough activities that could cause that site to be in danger of a hard impact against it in any way.

The medications he had to take to prevent a rejection needed to be taken precisely as directed, always the correct dose at the correct time. Certain foods were to be avoided that may cause the medicine to not work properly. A whole new diet was needed to ensure the new kidney stayed healthy and to reduce the chances of infection or rejection.

A journal was to be kept charting temperature, blood pressure, weight, and medications taken each day and tracking the dose and the times taken for the doctor to review at each follow up appointment. This information would show if the many medications needed adjustment along the way (which they would need to be) to ensure they continued to work properly for each patient. The medications become part of the recipient's routine for life. The patient also will need to record how much he drinks and the amount of urine he passes each day for at least the first six weeks.

Doctors' visits and lab work are required one to two times a week at first, and even though they won't be as frequent as that, they will continue to be required also to keep track of important information to ensure there is not a chance of rejection.

There is so very much to be thankful for after a successful transplant, of course, but then again, the realization for a young 19-year-old son that life would be different in many ways too is difficult. A brotherly separation was taking place, and as the mother of twin sons, I knew it would be something to get used to. They always did everything together for so many years, like biking on long and hard bike trails, hiking, boating, skiing, skateboarding, playing soccer on the same teams, and more. My heart hurt for them.

Jason was heading off to college to begin figuring out what he wanted to do in life, and Jake was faced with taking time to recover and get used to a different way of life instead of being able to begin his college career with his brother.

It was a time of mixed emotions for all of us. It didn't seem fair in a way. Along with knowing he'd need another kidney transplant when the incurable disease destroyed his new kidney, it just didn't seem fair.

Even with so very much to be thankful for, we had conflicting thoughts and emotions to work through. We knew one day again there would be the wondering and waiting for another transplant needed for his life to continue. The when tried to take over my thoughts, but I had to stop, trust that God was in control, and remember it's His timing, and He knows the right time even in trials and sorrow. It wasn't for me to try to figure out. He had proved to always be with us in whatever we faced, so I could replace the thoughts of when with thoughts of joy and thanksgiving once again because our son was here with us and becoming healthier each day. He had been blessed with a renewed life.

How blessed I had been to be able to give him one of my kidneys so that could happen, and I knew that when another kidney was needed, God already provided that need with his twin brother who would be able to be the donor.

The kidney I gave Jake lasted seventeen years, and then Jason was more than willing to give Jake a second kidney that is still working strong for Jake. It's giving him more life again. He's feeling good and enjoying being a father to his own son to love. Jason and I share the amazing and rewarding experience of donating a kidney to Jake. Being able to donate successfully to one in need is not only a gift to that person, but it's such a gift to the one giving. The love felt is like none other; the blessing is truly from God. I was so thankful I was a match to be able to do that for my son. Seeing my son, Jason, give his brother a kidney was so incredibly beautiful to witness. My heart was full because of the love they share, which was visible as they were preparing to go into the separate operating rooms. It was exactly the kind of love that God wants all of us to share and experience in our lives.

I sincerely pray that everyone who is able considers being an organ donor. I pray when you see a need, you will be tested to see if you could be the match needed for the opportunity to give a renewed life to a person in need. It is truly an amazing feeling to know you gave new health, love, and compassion to another person, whether it is family, friend, or stranger, and in return, you will feel the love and compassion and God's blessings upon you.

"Each one must give as he has decided in his heart, not reluctantly or under compulsion, for God loves a cheerful giver."
– 2 Corinthians 9:7 (ESV)

"This is my commandment, that you love one another as I have loved you."
– John 15:12 (ESV)

I can almost guarantee that each transplant donor and recipient will have a unique experience. Why does the proposed recipient need a transplant? What caused the person to discover he/she needed a transplant? Will the need be fulfilled by a living donor, or will the need be placed on a transplant list? The list will have people of all ages and from all walks in life. Where does the recipient live? Where does the donor live? Where will the surgery take place? Does the recipient have a loving family to support him/her? Have the recipient and the donor received the truth that they are a child of

God? Each one will have a story to share in one way or the other.

Lori shared when asked, "How have these experiences challenged and changed your faith in God?"

"Everyone will respond differently to things like this. Situations like this are never easy, and I do not think anyone can explain the whys. I would say that he/she needs to be encouraged to move on to hope and focus on the outcome. Express that this seems unfair, hard, sad, and worrisome. It is okay to feel this way. It challenges your faith; it brings up a million questions that cannot be answered no matter how much you ask, but one thing I know for sure is that no one can go through something like this alone. Find someone to talk to whether it is family, friends, strangers, ministers or professionals. People are there to listen. Don't keep it bottled up and carry the weight on your shoulders. If you are angry, be angry. If you are sad, or if you are worried, tell someone you are worried, but then move on to a positive attitude and find hope. Pray that all will be as it should be. Understand that the outcome will be what it should be no matter what. Accept it. You must dig deep and work at dealing with the situation from start to finish. Negativity will only make matters worse. Don't go down the rabbit hole that you cannot climb out of. If your family is around, please talk to each other, rely on one another, be brave for each other, love each other, and pray together. Balance each other out. Find time to laugh together, even in situations like these. This is what family is for. God is there; He understands what you are going through."

Yvette:

My hope and prayer are that by sharing this story, you will gain strength to face whatever your circumstance is in your transplant need. I pray for each of you who may read this because you are facing a need for a transplant even though I may never know you. God knows you, and He will hear my prayer for those in need. We are all brothers and sisters in Christ. We are family, and I want you to know God's love for you. His Word is the Light of the world, and He can be there with us through every minute of every journey we will travel when we accept Christ into our life and obey His Word. He wants the best for us when we do that, and He always gets us to the other side of any problems we may face.

The words from an old hymn by John H. Sammis, written in 1887, come to mind. I remember singing it when I was a child. It is a perfect reminder to follow so we can be at peace about whatever might happen in life:

"Trust and obey, for there's no other way
To be happy in Jesus, but to trust and obey!"

Bobbie:

I have not experienced anything like the day after my son's kidney donation surgery. The level of joy, excitement, anticipation, and love could not be contained, and it poured out into the hallways and rooms of everyone involved in this kidney donation process. The previous day I left my son in the hospital to rest, and when I returned, he was showered, shaved, up, and walking. He mentioned being inspired by a previous donor who had done the same after his/her surgery. My son said he tried taking one step forward, and if that went well, he would take another and another. He found his balance and strength and prepared to meet everyone involved in the donation process. I was excited and amazed. I was thankful as well because we had come so far and now we got to meet his recipient! I couldn't believe this was happening! I didn't know what to think at this point because this all seems so unbelievable.

The next thing I knew my son was standing next to his recipient who thought he was someone from the hospital or another family member because he had changed out of his gown and into street clothes. Only my son would draw such a reaction. Once the confusion was cleared up, the celebration began, and names and backgrounds were exchanged. Hugs were shared, as well as handshakes and high fives. We all were crying and cheering and so thankful everyone came through their surgeries as planned. Four surgeries were done the day before because of what's called a donor chain. Two people were walking and looking like nothing had happened. My son expressed feeling tired, but he wasn't showing it.

I look back on that experience and believe it couldn't have come out any better. My son has new friends for life, and I have new friends for life. Bonds were made that day in the hallway of MUSC that will not be broken or forgotten—all because of a sticker on the back of a car.

George:

Throughout preparation for kidney donation surgery, the nurses and support staff would share stories of how donors recovered from surgery. Some donors would stay an extra day or two in the hospital to help manage pain. Others would be up and walking the next morning ready to go. I wanted to be up, dressed, and walking the next morning, but most of all, I looked forward to meeting everyone involved in the kidney donation chain. Our plan was to meet around 11 AM, and I couldn't wait. I had no idea who would receive my kidney and now the surgeries were complete and the time had come to find out! By the grace of God, we all came through our surgeries without issue, and we all wanted to meet each other. Somehow, I had also managed to shower and get dressed before our meeting. If you had asked me several hours before 11 AM that day, I would have said no way but my strength and resolve quickly grew as 11 AM came closer.

I walked into the hallway a little after 11 AM toward a group of people. Two were in hospital gowns, and the rest were in regular clothes. My mother came with me as well. When I used to run marathons, she would travel with me to many of them and meet me at the finish line. I am grateful she was able to be with me at this finish line too. I met my recipient, and we celebrated! Together we rang the celebration bell in the hallway at least six or seven times. We cheered and cried tears of joy. Our doubts in the process had been defeated as we got to embrace each other and thank God for His faithfulness. We were now a family of four, plus all our supporting family and friends, and we spent the next hour getting to know each other. We gathered in the room of one of the recipients and had the opportunity to sign a special pillow MUSC had given to each of us. We wrote notes of encouragement and thanks to each other as we passed them around the room. This experience was one of the most precious times in my life, and I don't think I have ever seen so many people in one hospital room. I have my pillow to this day with the notes preserved, as well as when they were written. I think I was supposed to use the pillow more than I did, but I didn't want the notes to smear!

1 Corinthians 6:20 (NKJV) says, "For you were bought at a price; therefore, glorify God in your body and in your spirit, which are God's." The context of this verse comes from the apostle Paul writing to the Corinthians about the sexual immorality taking place among them. This verse is a reminder of the work Jesus did on the cross for humanity. Jesus died for the life change of believers. Through faith in Christ, your life will change and the change comes from the work of God. We have a responsibility to release our life and actions to God so we may live for God, and when we live for God, we bring change to others as well. You are here for reasons that are beyond your own, and your purpose is greater than you can think or imagine. You are here to make a difference, and through faith in Jesus, you are making a difference.

To make a difference in the name of Jesus, you must release your rights of how the difference looks to God. Trust in God to do the work and reveal your path to you, and be willing to take steps of faith along the way. When your steps of faith don't go how you had hoped they would go, keep moving forward and don't give up! Remember God maintains responsibility for the outcome, and our role is to be obedient. God is able and can handle the outcomes and we are to be considerate, courageous, and not callous. God is Creator and Builder, and we are created in His image. Through revelation in who we are through Christ, we too become creators and builders in the kingdom of God. Now is the time to build and continue to build and not because we have to but because we get to!

God's grace covers your mistakes and will bridge the gaps in what you think you lack. Remember this doesn't mean we do whatever we desire and act in a callous manner, but it does mean we take risks. We are called to do things that are greater than ourselves because God wants us to see His glory within the building. Be courageous, consider your family and friends, ask questions, discuss your ideas, and most of all, trust in God. The life of a Christian should be the most exciting experience on this earth. Christians are here to share the light of the world and bring the light to dark places. We are here to help. Finding out how you are called to help requires you to explore and gain experience through trial and error. You will take steps of faith that will end up in results that may disappoint you. To the world you may look like a failure, but remember God is working through you, and you are not working for God. Continue to release your rights to results to God and rejoice in His renewed mercy and compassion every day. The end of Romans 8 (NKJV) says, "Nothing separates us from the love of God." Your failures or omissions or doubts do not separate you from God's love. Return to Him in faith through Christ and continue to move forward.

Once I thought I was called to be a foster parent. In 2017, I went through an exhaustive process including in depth interviews, home studies, and hours of training. I believed God was calling me into this and was trusting in Him to provide what I would need to be a foster parent. My family was not enthusiastic about my endeavor. I wasn't sure how I was going to do this, but I began to work through the process to make it happen. I changed my work schedule, did some light remodeling of my house, and prepared as best I could to welcome a child into my home. My license came through, and I received a placement. In those first few days, I realized how under qualified I was for this calling. I had help, but I struggled. I became frustrated because I hadn't fully released my rights to the outcome to God. I had ideas and visions that were not my own, and when I got angry and frustrated, I began to want to give up.

After about three weeks, I did and felt horrible about doing so, but I thought it was best for my current situation. I did beat myself up emotionally and felt like I had failed God, but through the love and encouragement of my family and friends, I realized that I was still standing, and today is a new day. So, I got up and kept moving forward. I didn't have another foster placement, but not too long after this, my daughters came back to live with me! I hadn't even thought about that happening, but all the preparations I made for becoming a foster parent had helped me to be ready for my daughters to live with me. If I hadn't gone through the preparations to become a foster parent, would they still have come to live with me? Maybe, but I do know that everything I went through in becoming a foster parent and what I went through as a foster parent revealed things I needed to work on within myself to be a better parent. The work continues to this day as well. God wants to grow us every day. Don't give up, and remember we all fall short of the glory of God. We need His grace, and He has given His grace to us. Learn from your mistakes, try not to repeat them, and be bold for the building of the kingdom of God. You are here to make a difference. God gives us resources so we may live and provide for our families.

Our resources may look like money, health, wisdom, time, etc. and since God has given them to us, may we also make them available for His use. I am not saying God wants you to give away everything you have worked for, but God does want you to hold onto them loosely. May we never forget that all things are possible for God, and may you be encouraged to know that if you were called to give away a lifetime of work, health, and achievement for the purposes of God, that God can restore all that has been given and more in the twinkling of an eye. Your calls from God will most often not make sense, and the path may be longer than you expected, but always remember Ephesians 3:20 tells us that God can do more than we think or imagine. I don't know about you, but I want to continue to be a part of the building of the kingdom of God. Let's stay engaged with God, read His Word, live to be an example of Jesus, and listen to the Holy Spirit.

A Prayer for Post Op Life:

May we thank God through Jesus Christ that our salvation comes not from works but from the grace of God through Jesus Christ! I want to encourage you through the words of Jesus in Matthew 7:21-23 (NKJV):

> *"Not everyone who says to Me, 'Lord, Lord,' shall enter*
> *the kingdom of heaven, but he who does the will of*
> *My Father in heaven. Many will say to Me in that day,*

'Lord, Lord, have we not prophesied in Your name, cast out demons in Your name, and done many wonders in Your name?' And then I will declare to them, 'I never knew you; depart from Me, you who practice lawlessness!'"

While this word may be more terrifying than encouraging on the surface, I hope you'll hear the heart of God. Trust in the finished work of Jesus and His righteousness for your salvation and not the work of your hands. Acts 17:30-31 (NKJV) says, ***"Truly, these times of ignorance God overlooked, but now commands all men everywhere to repent, because He has appointed a day on which He will judge the world in righteousness by the Man whom He has ordained. He has given assurance of this to all by raising Him from the dead."*** Jesus is the one who has died, been raised, and now lives with our Father in heaven. Receive the works of Jesus first and then go to work. Please do not make the mistake of those in Matthew 7 and attempt to work your way to God. God has come to you through faith in Jesus Christ. May the love you have for the saving work of Jesus Christ lead your heart, fill your mind, and guide your hands and feet.

The apostle Paul furthers this revelation by writing Ephesians 2:10 (NKJV), ***"For we are His workmanship, created in Christ Jesus for good works, which God prepared beforehand that we should walk in them."*** May your faith in Jesus Christ be your starting point for every good work and may His presence within you through the Holy Spirit sustain you through the steps and time.

Thank you, Lord, for the good works that have been given to us through the fullness of your mercy and grace! May our continued motivation for greater works be love for You and each other. May we not tire in our generosity and be patient through prayer towards opportunities of your grace. May we be led by the Holy Spirit and not feel burdened by continued labors, but continually rejoice in the opportunity to serve. Father, we acknowledge the truth that we are here to work, not for salvation, but for others to hear, see and receive the love you have for them in Jesus. You have given us the anointing of faith, hope, and love by Your Holy Spirit and may this anointing not be in vain through our lives. Your word says love never fails so may we *not fail to love even when it seems like evil prevails. Revelation 12:11 (NKJV) says, "**And they conquered him by the blood of the Lamb and by the word of their testimony, for they loved not their lives even unto death.**" I pray for boldness in sharing all the goodness You have blessed us with as Your children. May our testimony be used to encourage others into faith in God through Jesus Christ and to never give up on the grace You have given and the promises You have spoken.*

*1 Thessalonians 4:15-18 (NKJV) says, "**For this we say to you by the word of the Lord, that we who are alive and remain until the coming of the Lord will by no means precede those who are asleep. For the Lord Himself will descend from heaven with a shout, with the voice of an archangel, and with the trumpet of God. And the dead in Christ will rise first. Then we who are alive and remain shall be caught up together with them in the clouds to meet the Lord in the air. And thus we shall always be with the Lord. Therefore comfort one another with these words.**" We shall always be with the Lord through faith in Jesus Christ. May you be encouraged! Amen.*

About the Authors...

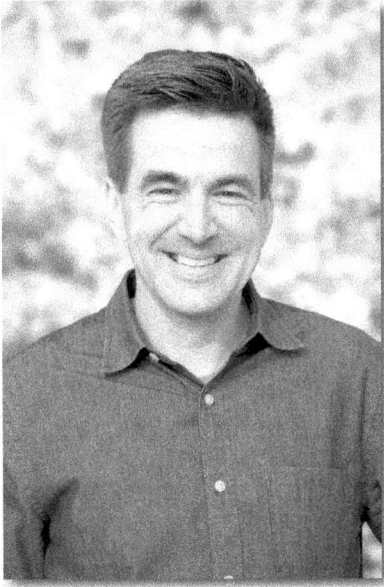

George Hansen became a living organ donor in the fall of 2022. Since donating his kidney, George's passion to help those on the transplant waiting list has not diminished. George hopes that by sharing his story alongside Yvette Kilgore, more people will be encouraged to donate. While the process to become a living donor can be challenging, the procedures have been built upon decades of experience and research. George wants those in similar circumstances to understand they are not alone and hopes every reader asks throughout these stories, "If God has done it for him/her, then why wouldn't He help me too?"

Since donating in 2022, George has experienced a full recovery and enjoys the many activities he participated in before surgery. George continues to share his talents and giftings to help people remain encouraged in the goodness of God because he has been encouraged through his own blessings from God. George has two wonderful, loving, and creative daughters and currently lives in Myrtle Beach, South Carolina.

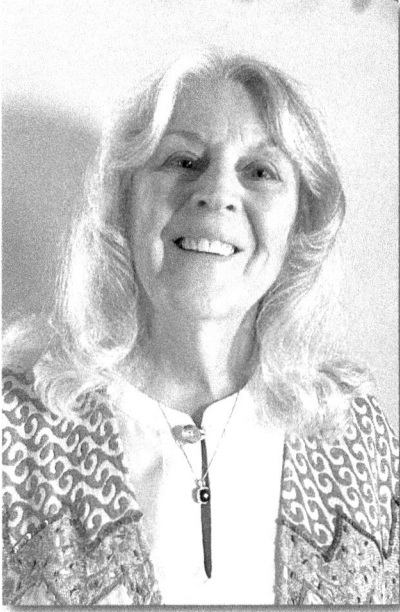

Yvette and her husband Gary live in Myrtle Beach, South Carolina. They have lived in Ohio; Ankara, Turkey; California; North Carolina; and South Carolina and have been blessed to travel to many countries in this beautiful world. They are proud parents of one daughter, two sons, and five grandchildren.

Yvette felt inspired to share in her first book, *Sunsets After The Storms*, her life experiences, the good and the bad. She told others about the love of God and how He led her to the other side of whatever came her way, including the loss of their home, sickness leading to organ transplants, losing faith, and wanting to give up. But by God's mercy and grace, she found an even stronger faith in Jesus.

These collective experiences and her faith in Jesus as her Lord and Savior enabled her to be a part of this book, *Patience for the Patient*, written with George Hansen. Life is good because God is good.

The Faces of This Book

We hope these images provide you, the reader, with a tangible connection to the stories within this book; going beyond just names into real, recognizable individuals.

It is our hope that you engage with the humanity behind the experiences; reminding you that each donor and recipient is a person with their own life, struggles, and emotions. Remember you are not alone in your experience.

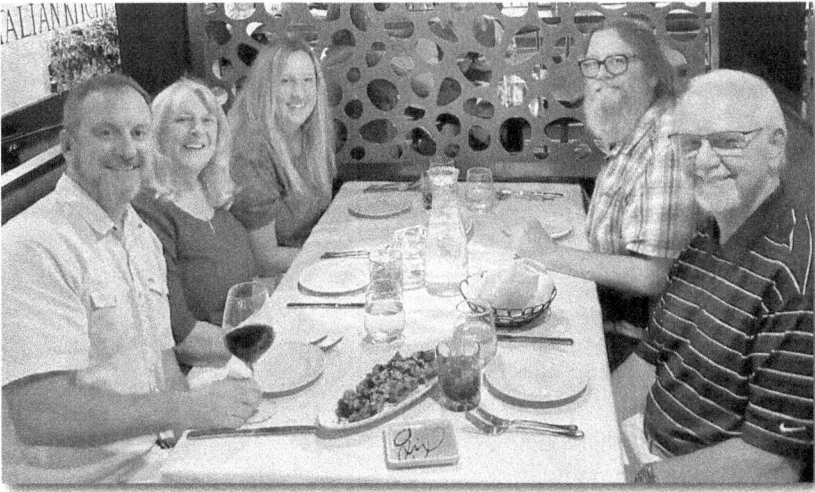

Yvette's family: from left to right: Jason, Yvette, Lori, Jake, and Gary.

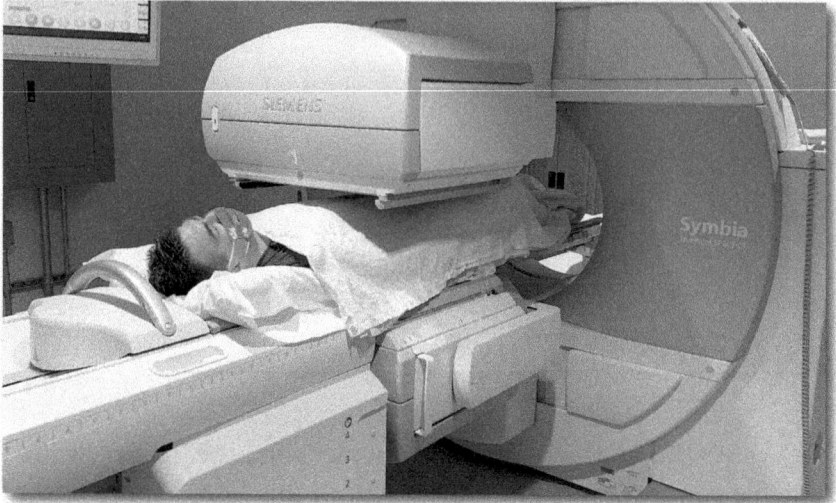

George is undergoing kidney function testing for clearance to become a living donor in the spring of 2021.

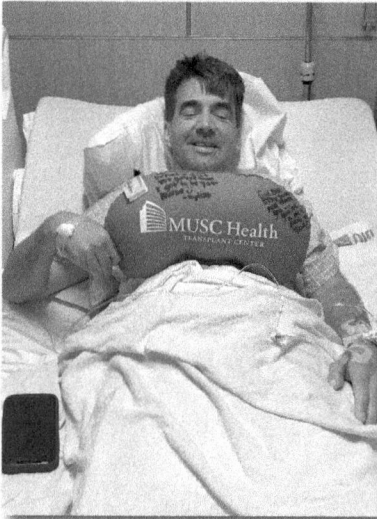

George in bed recovering from surgery. He is holding the pillow MUSC gives to recipients and donors after surgery to help with recovery. Traditionally doctors, nurses, recipients and donors will sign the pillow.

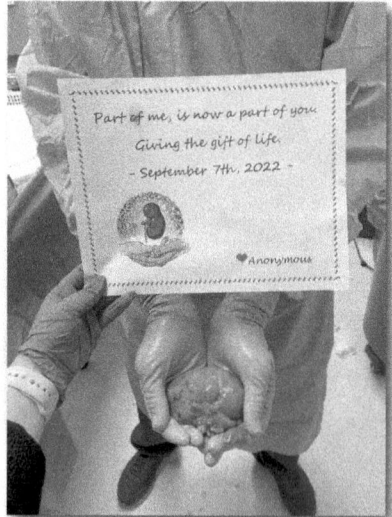

George's kidney in the operating room.

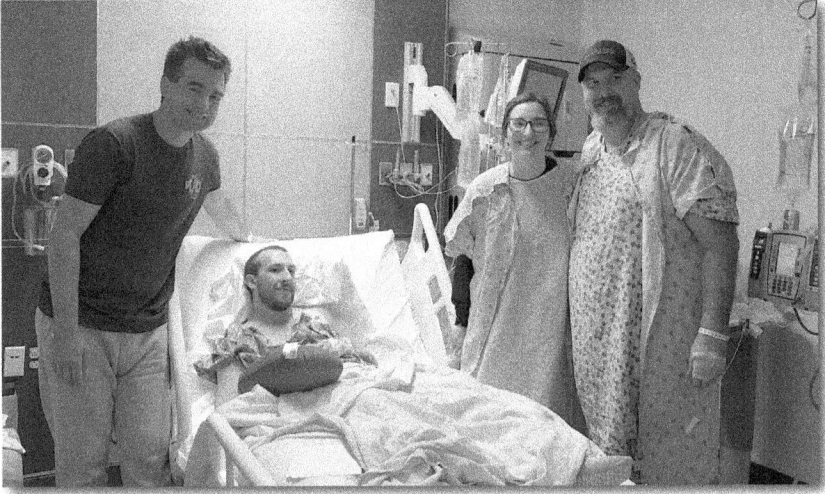

From right to left: Matt King, Jessica King, Nicholas Bland, and George Hansen. Matt King is George's recipient. Jessica King donated to Nicholas Bland. All 4 surgeries happened the same day and this photo is from the meet and greet the day after the surgeries.

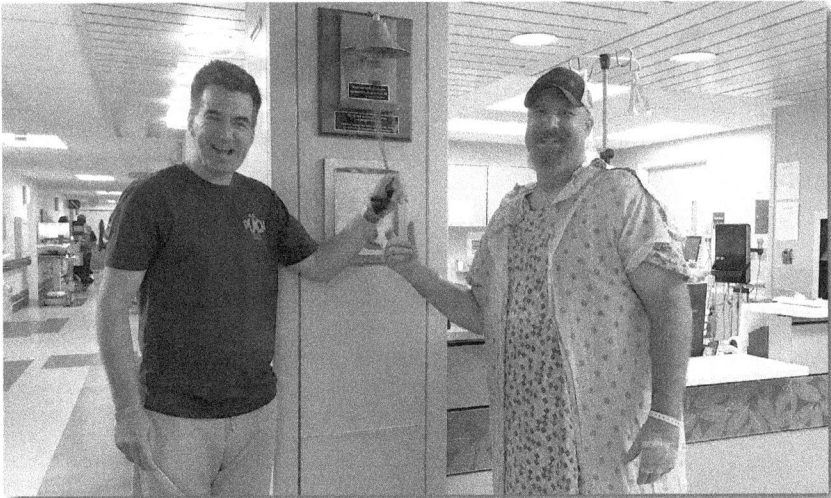

Matt King and George ringing the "victory" bell at MUSC the day after surgery.

Resources

If you have been encouraged through the stories of this book and would like more information about becoming a living donor in South Carolina, please contact the MUSC Living Donor Team in Charleston, SC, at 843-792-5097. More information is also available online.

https://muschealth.org/medical-services/transplant/living-donation

You may also find more information about programs throughout the United States here

https://www.organdonor.gov/learn/process/living-donation

Help is also available for living donors to cover travel expenses and loss of work wages through the organ donation process. Please contact the National Living Donor Assistance Center (NLDAC) at 888-870-5002 and online

https://www.livingdonorassistance.org

If you are waiting for a kidney transplant and would like to talk with others who have experienced a similar trial, contact the Transplant Talk Mentor Project. Transplant Talk was founded by organ donation recipients, and their goal is to help patients navigate the transplant path with comfort and encouragement. Transplant Talk also helps care givers of recipient patients as well. For more information, visit them online

https://transplanttalksc.org

The next step website brings living organ donation resources together on one website and also gives living organ donors the opportunity to share their story to help encourage others. For more info, visit

https://www.nextstepnextone.com/

Additional information is available at the National Kidney Foundation, http://www.kidney.org. "One in three Americans are at-risk for kidney disease," and at UNOS (United Network for Organ Sharing), http://www.unos.org, According to the UNOS (United Network for Organ Sharing), "6,466 people became living donors in 2022, fewer than 2021." And also, "The need is real. Another person is added to the waiting list every nine minutes."